Understanding
Osteoporosis

Also by Naheed Ali

Understanding Hepatitis: An Introduction for Patients and Caregivers

Understanding Fibromyalgia: An Introduction for Patients and Caregivers

Understanding Chronic Fatigue Syndrome: An Introduction for Patients and Caregivers

Understanding Lung Cancer: An Introduction for Patients and Caregivers

Understanding Celiac Disease: An Introduction for Patients and Caregivers

Understanding Alzheimer's: An Introduction for Patients and Caregivers

Understanding Parkinson's Disease: An Introduction for Patients and Caregivers

The Obesity Reality: A Comprehensive Approach to a Growing Problem

Arthritis and You: A Comprehensive Digest for Patients and Caregivers

Diabetes and You: A Comprehensive, Holistic Approach

UNDERSTANDING
OSTEOPOROSIS
An Introduction for Patients and Caregivers

NAHEED ALI

ROWMAN & LITTLEFIELD
Lanham • Boulder • New York • London

Published by Rowman & Littlefield
An imprint of The Rowman & Littlefield Publishing Group, Inc.
4501 Forbes Boulevard, Suite 200, Lanham, Maryland 20706
www.rowman.com

86-90 Paul Street, London EC2A 4NE

British Library Cataloguing in Publication Information Available

Library of Congress Cataloging-in-Publication Data Is Available

ISBN: 978-1-5381-6814-1 (cloth: alk. paper)
ISBN: 978-1-5381-6815-8 (electronic)

∞™ The paper used in this publication meets the minimum requirements of American National Standard for Information Sciences—Permanence of Paper for Printed Library Materials, ANSI/NISO Z39.48-1992.

To my mother

Disclaimer

This book is for reference only. It is not intended as a medical manual, and the data presented here are meant to assist the reader in making informed choices regarding wellness. This book is not a replacement for treatment(s) that the reader's personal physician may have suggested. If the reader believes he or she is experiencing a medical issue, then professional medical help is recommended. Mention of particular products, companies, or authorities in this book does not entail endorsement by the publisher or author.

Contents

CONTENTS

Author's Note

This book is not meant for medical professionals; however, the nonmedical reader may encounter advanced medical terminology throughout the writing. This is often necessary for the intended comprehensive review of the subject and because certain medical concepts necessitate clarification well beyond a modest introduction.

Preface

A normal bone is made up of various collagen, proteins, and calcium. It has two types: cortical bone, which makes up the body or shaft of the long bones, and trabecular bone, which can be found on the knoblike ends of the long bones, vertebrae, wrists, feet, and the iliac crest of the pelvis, the protruding bone that can be felt at the hips.[1]

Introduction to Osteoporosis

Osteoporosis, or OP, is a medical condition where the bones become fragile and brittle due to a decrease in density. It is characterized by bones that have large, spongy pores that are too far apart when seen through a microscope. Because these pores are not as compact as before, fractures can most likely occur.[2]

There are two types of OP: postmenopausal or estrogen/androgen deficient (type 1), and age-related (type 2) OP. In type 1 OP, caused by the reduction of sex hormones due to menopause, patients are commonly women. Men may also experience type 1 OP if their androgen levels have declined over the years. The fracture site is placed primarily at the vertebrae, which is composed of trabecular bones, but can also affect the ribs, pelvis, and femur.[3]

Type 2 OP affects all genders since the process of replacing old bone cells with new ones declines with age. Most patients develop the disorder by age 65. Because it affects both trabecular and cortical bones, fractures can happen in any part of the skeletal system.[4]

THE IMPORTANCE OF READING ABOUT OSTEOPOROSIS

Osteoporosis affects quality of life of senior citizen patients, not to mention the medical bills associated with fixing a bone structure: A medical procedure to ease the pain of a herniated disc, a slip of the cushion bone where the spine is connected, costs around $20,000–$50,000 without insurance.[5]

If diagnosed early on, OP patients can seek treatment that can slow down disease progression. However, nothing beats prevention, especially if it can be easily done through simple lifestyle changes that can be made today.[6]

SIGNIFICANCE OF A COMPREHENSIVE APPROACH TO OSTEOPOROSIS

Women develop loss of bone density as they reach their late 20s. Based on the statistics provided by National Institute of Arthritis and Musculoskeletal and Skin Diseases, one out of two women over 50 will develop an OP-related fracture in their lifetime.[7]

This does not mean that men do not develop OP. Physicians are less likely to diagnose elderly men even after exhibiting an OP-related fracture due to the prejudice that it only happens to women. Furthermore, costs of treating OP in men are expected to rise to around half of those associated with treating women by 2030.[8]

DIAGNOSING OSTEOPOROSIS

Because the diagnosis of osteoporosis is relatively straightforward, although lacking in major practical advancement in recent times beyond bone density assessment, the science of asserting whether a person has osteoporosis will be covered in brief at this time. Osteoporosis is diagnosed through a bone mineral density (BMD) test using dual-energy X-ray absorptiometry (DXA). The results are interpreted using T-scores and are compared to the standards provided by the World Health Organization (WHO):

- If the T-score is -1.0 or above, the patient has normal bone mineral density.
- If the T-score is between -1.0 and -2.5, the patient has osteopenia, another bone disorder characterized by a slightly less dense bone density but not classified as OP.
- If the T-score is -2.5 or below, the patient has OP.[9]

The T-scores were obtained by examining a sample of white postmenopausal women in the early 1990s. Because of this, they cannot be loosely applied to other races or even to men. Thus, a group of researchers reevaluated the WHO standards and developed the Fracture Risk Assessment Tool (FRAX), a standard used to determine the patient's 10-year probability of fracture by considering other factors that can contribute to OP risk: the country where the patient came from, body mass index (BMI), and unfavorable habits such as excessive alcohol intake and smoking, among others.[10]

However, there are places around the world that have no access to central DXA screening. In this case, a peripheral screening test is done, which measures the BMD of the finger, wrist, heel, or lower arm to determine if the patient needs further testing. These tests, along with central DXA at the radius bone found in the forearm, are also given to patients weighing 300 pounds or more, since machines are not able to detect the hip and spine on obese patients.[11]

I
BASIC PICTURE

I

History of Osteoporosis

THERE IS NO RECORD OF HOW BONE DISORDERS FIRST APPEARED in known history. However, the first diagnosed bone disorder is achondroplasia, a type of disproportionate dwarfism characterized by a short stature even in adulthood (about four feet at most), a large head in proportion to the length of arms and legs, a prominent forehead, and a flat nose. Early scientists believed the condition was brought about by "weak semen," when in truth, it is brought about by a mutation in the FGFR3 gene, which is responsible for skeletal growth and development. Because of their unusual appearance, people with achondroplasia have been the subject of folklore and stories made by poets and writers, as evidenced by the fairy tale *Gulliver's Travels.* They could also be seen as a form of entertainment in circuses and carnivals, performing tricks and acts that gave their stature an advantage. Despite their seemingly glamorous popularity, sadly, most of them were shunned by society, making research related to their disease difficult to obtain. Myth and speculation became the substitute for sound truth.[1]

BRIEF HISTORY OF BONE DISORDERS IN GENERAL

Sometime in 1892, German pathologist Eduard Kaufmann, using illustrations and write-ups, discussed the skeletal diseases commonly found in infants. He recognized the differences in the various bone disorders afflicted by the newborns and used illustrations he made to prove and explain his point. Achondroplasia was one of his discoveries, although the cause of the disease at the genetic level was yet to be discovered during his lifetime. His study of the pathology of these bone disorders and the later development of X-rays became the foundation of bone disorder diagnosis as it is today.[2]

In 1785, the mechanism of the X-ray, a widely used method to diagnose bone disorders, was discovered, albeit unknowingly, by William Morgan, who published a paper with the Royal Society of London about a glow produced by X-rays when electric currents passed through a vacuum tube. However, it was not until William Röntgen studied the mechanism discovered by Morgan and further developed it in 1895 that X-rays were officially used by the public. While Röntgen is the first person to discover the possible role of X-rays in the medical field by photographing his wife's hand and seeing her bones underneath the flesh, it was actually John Hall-Edwards who first used them in clinical circumstances. Hall-Edwards used X-rays to find and examine a needle left stuck in the hand of one of his associates; he was also the first to radiograph (produce pictures by X-rays or other body imaging equipment) the spine and to use the machine during a surgical procedure. X-rays later paved the way for the development of other radiologic equipment for medical purposes.[3]

It is only after World War II that biochemistry and genetics flourished along with the medical sciences. With the help of X-rays and clinical findings, bone disorders were slowly being discovered by physicians and scientists. The discovery of how lifestyle and genetics play a role in the development of bone disorders led to study and observation by researchers that has helped the medical community in diagnosing and treating this type of disease.[4]

HISTORY OF OSTEOPOROSIS

Osteoporosis was first observed by anthropologists on the skeletal remains of early humans. Radiographs of the bones indicated that they exhibited bone density loss and other OP-related changes, including a porous, spongelike appearance in the knobs. The anthropologists deduced that this was caused by the heavy labor associated with agriculture and the chronic malnutrition rampant in the area where the bones were found. The remains showed that OP has been around long before doctors and scientists became aware of it. In Egypt, paleopathologists have observed porotic (with holes) bones on Egyptian mummies. Even today, they are still finding out the cause of osteoporosis in the past with the hope that it can help improve current interventions being employed to prevent and treat OP.[5]

It was in the eighteenth century that the English surgeon John Hunter discovered bone remodeling. He observed that as soon as new bone is introduced, the old one is destroyed or reabsorbed by the new one. Even though this process is known to be the foundation of OP treatment, the concept of bone remodeling and its relationship to OP was not established until more than a hundred years after he died later.[6]

Later on, Astley Cooper, a pathologist and sergeant surgeon of Queen Victoria, discovered the relationship of bone density loss to age and fracture risk, discussed in his book *Dislocations and Fractures*, published in 1882. By this time, the medical community had already recognized that the disease favored elderly women more than men, thereby offering traction to the wheel of unspoken prejudice that made OP underdiagnosed and undertreated in men.[7]

It didn't help that 50 years later, the American endocrinologist Fuller Albright discovered the role of menopause on the development of OP. After all, it is rare to find men who experience low androgen levels as they age, and those who do often do not talk to their physicians about it. This leads to unsurprising statistics related to the underdiagnosis and undertreatment of OP in their sex.[8]

Albright's discovery of the relationship between OP and menopause was duly noted by the medical community. Later on, he started using estrogen to treat women with the disorder. Unfortunately, the treatment is capable only of preventing or possibly delaying the progress of the disease. During Albright's time, there were no instruments invented yet that were capable of detecting the early signs of OP, making it difficult to determine when to start treatment using estrogen therapy.[9]

With this problem in mind, scientists developed more sensitive machines that could detect bone loss in its early stages. One of these instruments is a densitometer, a device that measures bone density by dispatching concentrated energy through the skin all the way to the bones of the wrists, hand, spine, hip, knee, and other body parts heavily prone to OP-related fractures. By measuring the intensity of the emitted energy, doctors can determine how dense or porous the specific bone. Densitometers were later refined into what is now collectively called DXA.[10]

Pharmacology also has its own contribution to the treatment of OP. A Swiss researcher named Herbert Fleisch discovered that biphosphonates can treat and slow down the progression of bone loss by prohibiting the death, or apoptosis, of old bone cells. The full extent of the drug and others that were discovered to lower the risk of OP will be discussed later in this book.[11]

As numbers of afflicted patients continued to grow through the years, the National Institutes of Health (NIH) named the disease a national health threat in 1984 and informed the general public how it can be prevented. New and improved treatments and other preventive measures are continuously being explored by researchers even today.[12]

HOW AND WHEN THE TERM *OSTEOPOROSIS* CAME TO BE

Caregivers should note that the term osteoporosis comes from the Greek word "osteo," meaning bone, and "poros," meaning pore. The coining of the term and the earliest observation of the pathological signs and symptoms of the disease is attributed to the French pathologist Jean Lobstein, who witnessed his patients exhibiting the porotic bones associated with OP in 1883. Lobstein was able to observe fully the debilitating disease while performing an autopsy on a 65-year-old man whose bones softened when he was eighteen years old and who ended up with tumors. In modern medicine, this condition can be called juvenile osteoporosis, a type of OP that afflicts children and adolescents rather enigmatically. After treating the man, Lobstein noticed that the affected bones became normal once they reabsorbed and healed as one, a phenomenon that had been previously observed by Hunter. Lobstein later published a journal article discussing the occurrence and used the term "osteoporosis" to describe the large porosity he has seen in the man's bones. The word spread like wildfire in medical circles, earning it a spot in the German dictionary by the late 1930s.[13]

ANALYSIS

Osteoporosis and bone disorders in general are being approached by experts in an increasingly effective manner. Owing to the efforts of the early pathologists, physicians, and researchers, diagnosis and treatment of the disease is becoming more refined and sophisticated than ever. Sadly, the number of people who experience the debilitating disease is steadily rising despite the continuous struggle to contain it.[14]

2

Osteoporosis around the World

OSTEOPOROSIS IS A WIDE-REACHING HEALTH PROBLEM, WITH estimates supporting claims that OP-related fractures happen every three seconds in real time. One in three women may experience these fractures in their lifetime, while one out of five men can develop it after reaching 50. Despite the gap, men have higher mortality rates than women related to OP due to the underdiagnosis and undertreatment of the disease in men. With its reputation as an imminent national threat, researchers continue to observe the trends related to OP and devise ways to make the instances of underdiagnosis and undertreatment of OP shrink. Their understanding of the statistics helps them to grasp whether the current interventions are paying off or are in need of improvement.[1]

OSTEOPOROSIS IN THE UNITED STATES

In the United States alone, roughly half a million Americans are at risk for OP-related fractures in their lifetime, particularly men and women ages 50 and up. If current trends continue, the affected population will increase substantially. Women, regardless of age and culture, are still most affected by the disease. In 2010, the prevalence of OP among women age 50 was three times higher than that of men in the same age group. The gap continued to increase with age, up to age 80. Again, this does not mean that men do not die from the disease; in fact, by the age of 50, men's risk of developing OP is higher than that of developing prostate cancer. The best example of this phenomenon is seen in Sweden, where more hospital stays are attributed to OP-related fractures than to prostate cancer.[2]

Juvenile OP springs up during puberty due to unknown causes, although it is only seen in a small number of the population. There are some cases in which young patients experience permanent disability because of the disorder, such as kyphoscoliosis, or the curving of the upper spine and a compromised rib cage. While it may appear and then go away spontaneously, it is still essential that affected children be given proper treatment in order to prevent the disease from affecting their growth and development.[3]

When it comes to race, OP is indiscriminate, although some races have lower significant risk than the others, specifically African Americans and Hispanics. It is observed that those with the highest risk have Caucasian and Asian ancestry. Risk factors are significantly dissimilar across race and ethnicity, so clinical approaches vary as well.[4]

Asians. Asians share almost the same risk factors as Caucasians. In fact, being Asian heightens the risk (compared to other ethnicities) that an individual will develop OP by age 50. Despite this, postmenopausal Asian women have the lowest prevalence of OP-related fractures than other races, although vertebral fractures are as likely to happen in Asians as in Caucasians. Some researchers believe that this is because most Asian women have small frames and therefore lower bone density. However, the former does not always equate to the latter, at least in clinical settings. More than half of the cases of OP-related fractures don't exhibit low bone density, further emphasizing the fact that bone density should not be the sole basis in considering OP risk.[5]

African Americans. African American women generally have higher bone density than those of other races. Unfortunately, mortality rates due to hip fracture are notably higher in this group. African American women also experience longer than usual hospital stays after a fracture and are the most likely to be permanently disabled afterward. These results are supported by the fact that OP is underdiagnosed and undertreated in African Americans. What's more, their risk for hip fracture doubles every seven years, explaining the high mortality rates. Secondary osteoporosis, the type of OP that stems from a medical condition, can also be a culprit since some diseases for which African Americans have the most risk can affect the bone-remodeling mechanism.[6]

Hispanics. This data group comprises individuals with Mexican, Cuban, Puerto Rican, Dominican, South American, Spanish, and other Latino descent, making up about more than 12 million people in the United States. The prevalence of OP-related fractures in Hispanics varies depending on the fracture site. For example, compared to Caucasian patients, the prospect of hip fracture in this group is one-third lower, while radius fractures have almost the same prevalence as in Caucasians. Another possible risk factor that might increase the possibility of developing OP is the fact that Hispanics are more likely than Caucasians to develop diabetes, a medical condition that can greatly affect the bone mechanism due to hormonal changes. Studies also show that most Hispanics have low bone mass beginning from early childhood, but not so low that it can be classified as OP. Theoretically, this means Hispanics need to be more careful in adhering to lifestyle changes associated with decreasing OP risk.[7]

Concerning the four races that mainly dominate the US population: All of them consume less than the recommended amounts of calcium and vitamin D. Adults should receive 1,200–1,500 milligrams of calcium every day. Calcium makes up close to 100 percent of the bone structure, making it a vital weapon against OP. The lack of it in the people's diets greatly increases their predisposition to this bone disorder.[8]

Osteoporosis in Other Countries

It is estimated that by 2050, the prevalence of OP will continue to increase threefold in women and more than twofold in men compared to 1990 statistics. It doesn't help OP patients or caregivers that only one-third of vertebral fractures are reported and treated satisfactorily. Experiencing this type of OP-resultant fracture increases a patient's risk of developing another fracture in a different bone site within the span of one year. As with the races and ethnicities, a varied approach to OP treatment is required for different countries on the basis of the resources available and the risk factors unique to their own cultures.[9]

Europe. The primary obstacle in OP diagnosis and treatment in Europe is limited resources, ranging from the unavailability of densitometers in primary care hospitals and lack of staff and medical professionals trained to perform the BMD procedure to a low overall healthcare budget. By 2025, WHO expects the number of OP patients to increase by 25 percent compared to 2010. In Sweden alone, the mortality rate for OP-related complications is the same as that of breast cancer, and the impact it makes on the patient's quality of life is greater than all cancers combined. In the nation of Georgia, only a quarter of the population with OP actually seek treatment and hospitalization. The medical costs incurred by OP in Swiss patients are significantly higher than those for heart disease, cancer, and chronic obstructive pulmonary disease. Denmark estimates that with the nation's current rates of OP, they could spend more than $1 billion (US) on treatment by 2025. If left unchecked, the bone disorder can seriously ravage the economy of the European Union.[10]

Canada. In Canada, one in four women and men over 50 are afflicted with OP and have experienced vertebral fracture once in their lifetime. The health sector expects that the incidence of OP in Canada will quadruple from the current rates soon.[11]

Latin America. It is estimated that, compared to 1990 rates, the incidence of OP in people ages 50–64 will increase by more than 300 percent by 2050 on the whole continent, all of which would cost more than $10 billion (US). In Argentina, healthcare centers treat close to 100 OP-related fractures each day. Hospitalization costs close to $200 million each year. In Brazil, one out of 17 residents has osteoporosis. Only one in three of them are diagnosed and only one out of five are actually treated. The disease costs them more than $5 million annually. In Mexico, one out of four has either osteopenia or osteoporosis.[12]

Middle East and Africa. Despite the abundance of natural sunlight in the Middle East and Africa, vitamin D intake is markedly low, making rickets a common illness. This is exacerbated by the fact that in most of the Middle East, women go out only in complete covering, greatly reducing their chances of soaking in the vitamin D that comes from the sun. Vitamin D also aids in bone remodeling and metabolism; hence, low levels of vitamin D increase the risk of developing OP in the long run. Unfortunately, diagnosis is next to impossible because DXA machines are scarce. In Morocco, there were times when more than 1 million were sharing the use of just one DXA machine. Lebanese women develop OP much younger than their Western counterparts, and more than 50 percent of them have osteopenia. With cultural and lifestyle factors in play, it is highly likely that it would advance into osteoporosis. In Syria, less than a quarter of those with OP are able to see and be treated by a doctor due to a dearth of funds and the tense political climate. In a study made in a sample of children living in Qatar, more than half have vitamin D deficiency, most in their preteen and adolescent stages.[13]

Asia. It is estimated by the year 2050, half of the worldwide cases of OP-related fractures will come from Asia. Because of their cultural practices, most OP patients are left undiagnosed and untreated even after they experience OP-related fractures. In rural China, hip fractures are often treated at home using traditional Chinese medicine. Caregivers and healthcare professionals in most developing countries can't afford DXA machines; those that are available are usually located in the capital and urban cities. Thus, most undiagnosed OP cases are seen in rural areas, where Western medicine and proper treatment is not widely available. WHO also notes that almost all Asian countries exhibited low intake of calcium; most Asians consume only one-third of the recommended daily allowance. Most of the countries in South Asia also have high rates of vitamin D deficiency in all age groups and both sexes.[14]

Oceania. More than 2 million Australians have been diagnosed historically with either osteopenia or osteoporosis. This costs the government close to $8 billion (US) annually, with about $2 billion spent on direct costs such as medicines and surgery. New Zealand spends at least $2 billion every year for OP-related expenses, with a significant rise in overall costs projected in the next few years.[15]

ANALYSIS

Osteoporosis is a debilitating disease that can impact anyone, regardless of gender, race, and culture. It is more prevalent than cancer and heart disease combined. Not only does it affect the patient who has the disease, but the government shares the burden of treating and preventing the disease, often at a great cost. Despite the magnitude of the problem, there are ways to apprise the general public of the extent of OP worldwide.[16]

3

The Roles of Outpatient Physicians and Patients in Osteoporosis

Doctors are not always around to accommodate the growing number of OP patients. Thus, it is vital that patients know how to take care of themselves while not under the direct care of a physician. Regrettably, there is no one type of specialization that can treat OP; to manage treatment well, patients benefit from the expertise of specialists from an assortment of medical fields.[1]

Types of Outpatient Medical Specialties Involved in Osteoporosis

Internist. Internists specialize in internal medicine. They can diagnose and treat many diseases, including OP. They can also act as consultants to the other specialists when it comes to OP treatment.[2]

Endocrinologist. In some cases, OP is brought on by another medical condition involving hormones, for example, diabetes or hyperthyroidism. This is called secondary osteoporosis.

Endocrinologists ensure that patients with such metabolic disorders can keep the problem from affecting the bones. They can also provide hormonal therapy to primary OP patients.[3]

Rheumatologist. Rheumatologists are responsible for diagnosing and treating diseases related to the skeletal and muscular system. They are the perfect go-to for OP advice, although they cannot do it all on their own. They help patients get the necessary and relevant laboratory tests in order to know their risk for OP and other diseases.[4]

Radiologist. X-rays and other medical imaging methods are essential to knowing and observing the appearance of the bones before and after OP-related symptoms settle in. Radiologists ensure these results are obtained and properly interpreted so they can be used by the primary care physician.[5]

Geriatrician. Geriatricians focus on diseases and other issues related to the health of senior patients. They have a broad and deep knowledge of the process of aging, which gives them a crucial role in treating OP since most of the afflicted are in or approaching their senior years.[6]

Orthopedic surgeon. These surgeons are involved in the branch of medical science dealing with musculoskeletal diseases, mostly via surgical means. These doctors can, however, use both surgical and nonsurgical methods to treat OP.[7]

Physiatrist. After surgery, it is likely that the surgical site will have limited range of movement, either temporarily or permanently. Not to be confused with *psychiatrists*, physiatrists emphasize rehabilitation in patients who have undergone surgery and those who have had minor fractures to ensure that they still live happy, healthy lives despite their condition.[8]

Dietician. Clinical nutritionist-dieticians can assist patients in obtaining proper nutrition through diet and lifestyle changes. Depending on the risk or severity of OP, dieticians can recommend individualized nutritional care plans and follow up with patients to evaluate progress.[9]

Some experts identify OP as an "orphan disease" because it is contained and treated by not just one specialist but a host of them. Open communication, then, with the whole healthcare team is a must to ensure the patient survives and lives as normal a life as possible.[10]

A Typical Day for an Outpatient Doctor Treating Osteoporosis

Patients who don't know that OP involves various specialists understandably first consult their family doctor. This physician, a medical professional trained to be knowledgeable in a variety of clinical disorders, then explains the processes involved, including the assemblage of healthcare specialists who can assist. The family doctor provides referrals to the rheumatologist and endocrinologist to further examine the patient.[11]

Internally, the different body systems work in tandem to keep a human being alive. Internists recognize and study this close relationship to provide long-term, holistic, and systematic care and management both in a hospital and outpatient clinical setting for patients who are at risk of OP or for those who have undergone surgery to treat their fracture. Internists make sure that each OP treatment is done without jeopardizing another organ system, since their goal is to help patients recover and prevent further complications. Thus, constant communication and a good relationship must be nurtured with patients to encourage them to come and be checked repeatedly. Internists also communicate with other members of the healthcare team to understand what measures can be used to treat OP patients.[12]

Endocrinologists recommend specific tests with the goal of ruling out possible metabolic and hormonal factors associated with OP and, if possible, preventing it from getting worse. Depending on patients' medical history and family history, endocrinologists order blood tests to see the levels of hormones in the blood. For a patient at risk of diabetes, for example, the endocrinologist would order either an oral glucose tolerance test (OGTT) or fasting blood sugar test (FBS) to determine the level of insulin in the bloodstream. If the patient has a heart disease risk, the specialist may want complete blood count (CBC) data to see the patient's cholesterol levels among other indicators. Caregivers can assist with patient scheduling in this regard.[13]

Rheumatologists are also qualified to interpret BMD tests since OP is as much a part of the musculoskeletal system, considering the results to the clinical findings collected from the OP patient to provide the proper treatment and interventions suitable for the specific patient's condition. Long after the patient has gone home, the rheumatologist can and must continue to monitor and follow up for changes in terms of mobility and lifestyle management.[14]

The most common examination is the BMD test using a DXA, or DEXA, machine. Using a cautiously calibrated machine in order to obtain the most accurate results, radiologists can identify if a specific bone structure is at a high risk of experiencing fracture and whether a specific fracture is caused by OP. Studies have shown that OP was immediately proclaimed once the radiology report mentioned the presence of OP-related fractures, whether or not recommendation for treatment was to be made afterward. Radiologists are also able to interpret different body imaging results related to any particular disease.[15]

Most geriatricians work in nursing homes rather than in a hospital setting. Their typical day includes checking on their senior patients and monitoring their current situation. Although geriatricians' role may seem superfluous with that of physicians, their expertise in geriatric care makes them a vital part in the OP healthcare team. Numerous studies conclude that the combined efforts of orthopedic surgeons and geriatricians result in shorter hospital stays and lasting improvement in life and daily activities for OP patients despite the presence of a debilitating disease. It is highly recommended that elderly patients be attended by a geriatrician from the time they check in at the orthopedic ward until they go home to return to their life routines. Intervention by a geriatrician makes the treatment recommended by other healthcare providers more efficient.[16]

Medical leaders often think orthopedic surgeons must only be involved when an OP-related fracture transpires. The primary goal in the scope of surgical care, then, is to avoid the occurrence of another fracture that could further debilitate the life of the patient. Over the years, however, orthopedic surgeons have argued that they have a critical role in the clinical picture even before the occurrence of fracture in order to provide preventive measures, whether surgical or not. They won. Now, orthopedists are there to provide early interventions for patients at risk of developing OP, specifically postmenopausal women and the elderly. In this capacity, orthopedic surgeons meet with patients and members of the healthcare team to discuss the steps that can be taken to avoid the progression of the disease.[17]

Osteoporosis patients may have setbacks in figuring out how to become mobile and return to their daily activities following bone fracture and subsequent surgical treatment. Physiatrists help these patients undergo different rehabilitation programs to bring back mobility, or, if that is not possible, recommend alternative movements to the ones patients normally do. They also develop exercise and posture training for OP patients who have had a severed vertebra due to a fall or surgical complications. They are the specialists qualified to determine whether an OP patient can go back to sports or other rigorous activities requiring a lot of movement stress on already fragile bones.[18]

Osteoporosis can be averted by consuming enough calcium and vitamin D over a lifetime. Both nutrients are vital for bone remodeling and strengthening. Dieticians provide recommendations to OP patients as to which foods can provide these nutrients and how patients can maximize their intake. They also enlighten patients about the possible interactions of calcium and vitamin D on the food and drugs they are currently ingesting and provide adjustments to meet their needs. If an OP patient is lactose intolerant or hypersensitive to dairy—which is, of course, a rich source of calcium—a dietician can recommend suitable substitutes. In hospital settings, dieticians safeguard OP patients against malnutrition to (a) meet daily caloric, calcium, and vitamin D requirements and (b) guide them in continuing these dietary habits upon discharge from the inpatient environment (discussed in the following chapter).[19]

Osteoporosis aside, the specialists mentioned above treat multiple diagnoses simultaneously. The role of patients, therefore, is to be informed of the possible courses of action and to always heed the advice of their healthcare providers. Treatment and prevention are there only if the specialists and patients work hand in hand to stop the disease from affecting body systems beyond just the musculoskeletal.[20]

WHAT'S IT LIKE TO BE AN OSTEOPOROSIS OUTPATIENT?

From the patient's side of things, being passed around from one medical professional to another can be frustrating, not to mention the colossal medical costs that are part of the care package for the uninsured. The news of an OP diagnosis—or of any bone disorder for the matter—affects not only the physical facet of a person's life but also the emotional, mental, and social well-being. Thus, healthcare providers must also seek the help of patients' immediate family and loved ones in order to help them press on.[21]

One of the things OP patients worry about is the risk of dying due to the disease. In truth, it is not OP that kills per se; it is rather the complications that may develop alongside the condition. As mentioned in chapter 2, hip fractures have high mortality rates and are most commonly seen in African American women. However, men, regardless of race, are the most likely to die from hip fractures. To put the statistic in simple terms, nine out of 100 women in the typical OP age bracket are likely to die due to the medical obstacles brought by the fracture, usually in a span of one to two years after the bone breakage. For what it's worth, the somewhat good news is that hip fractures happen mostly to elderly patients, and younger people can avoid experiencing them with proper preventative measures.[22]

Death from a previous fracture at the wrist or leg is usually associated with some other preexisting medical condition rather than OP. This is why preexisting conditions must be ruled out by the endocrinologist to solve the puzzle early on and ensure a longer life for the patient.[23]

Life isn't so easy for OP patients after the fall, however. Many go through a lot of physical and mental agony due to the changes in appearance the disease brings. For example, height loss brought by a dowager's hump, the downward curvature of the upper spine, can be devastating to patients who were previously tall. Fewer than half the people who suffer a hip fracture are able to walk after the surgery. For patients who have been independent all their lives, this decrease in mobility may cause depression. They may also develop shame and guilt about burdening their loved ones with their care; loved ones who are unable to provide care themselves may be forced to move patients into a nursing home. Depression associated with OP will be discussed more thoroughly in chapter 8.[24]

Spinal fractures may also result in immobility, although not as severe as that involved with hip fractures. Osteoporosis patients who have had spinal fractures, however, suffer from tremendous pain in their lower back, an ailment that goes on for weeks or even months on end. Height loss is just one physical complication. Thankfully, the worst forms of spine fractures are well researched by the medical community, so specialists can provide adequate treatment to alleviate the pain and bring patients back to as normal a life as possible.[25]

In contrast, wrist fractures may not cause long-term disability but can still be troublesome, especially considering how frequently we use our hands for daily activities. Patients report of a lack of feeling in the hand when touched, a condition called carpal tunnel syndrome. Pain resurfaces, hand function is impaired, and arthritis ensues. Osteoporosis patients adjust to these changes, however, and symptoms usually last for only about six months.[26]

The emotional turmoil associated with OP-related fracture must also be given consideration, especially if the event brought debilitating effects. Anxiety attacks and fears about falling from a considerable height may result because patients are petrified about breaking another bone and plodding through the process of mending it all over again. Due to the height loss, outpatient OP sufferers who either have or lack very closely attached caregivers can experience low self-esteem and lack confidence to do errands on their own. Patients may not feel like going out and spending precious time with family and friends, leaving them feeling isolated and neglected. This feeling is only heightened once the family has decided that a nursing home is the best solution for a patient's care.[27]

Osteoporosis treatments cost a fortune, speaking figuratively, thereby adding a financial burden to the already long list of obstacles that OP patients, their families, and possibly their caregivers have to bear in order to nurse them back to health in an outpatient scenario. Unfortunately, some medical insurance plans do not cover close to 15 percent of the costs in managing OP symptoms, requiring patients and their families to pay out of pocket for these expenses. Another drawback families need to address is the caregiving needed for OP patients. Most families cannot afford a home nurse or caregiver, so adult family members may take turns caring for a patient. It's usually the young adults who are allotted this task, leading to decreased productivity and purchasing power for aspiring younger people; instead of working, they have to stay at home and tend to their sick loved ones.

Transferring a patient into a nursing home comes with a host of other financial considerations. Public facilities may be a minuscule amount cheaper than their private counterparts, but the level of care is often far lower.[28]

ANALYSIS

In addition to the effects of OP at the economic and national level, one must also consider the consequences it brings to individuals who suffer from OP in advance of, as well as after, the trip to the hospital. Facing the outcome of the medical condition to their physical health isn't enough; outpatients who have OP must also endure the intrinsic and extrinsic effects of this medical disorder. The family, too, are time and again dealing with difficulties caused by OP.[29]

4

The Role of Hospitals in Osteoporosis

In hospital organizations, OP patients are cared for in multiple ways, such as ensuring a comfortable environment, reducing pain, providing medical treatment for the specific condition, and providing a proper diet plan that aids in healing. Chiefs of respective departments within hospitals collaborate with their staff and nurses to help patients suffering from OP in a variety of inpatient health facilities. Health practitioners also ensure that individuals get appropriate diagnostic, treatment, and preventive services depending on the severity of each patient's OP.[1]

Hospitals are furnished with X-ray machines to view internal structures such as thinning bones to assess the progression rate of OP and determine the course of action to be taken. Patients and caregivers should also note that certain machines reveal (a) how brittle the bones are or if they might break at any time, (b) whether certain bone structures are still salvageable, and (c) if the individual ought to take more food rich in calcium and vitamin D. Osteoporosis sufferers are also given medication during the hospital stay to curb the rate of bone mass reduction.[2]

HOSPITALS CONTRIBUTE TO THE CARE OF OP SUFFERERS

Hospitals are where medical professionals raise awareness and educate the public on bone diseases. Hospitals also evaluate and monitor the health outcomes of people in the community for the presence of those with bone diseases. The most significant role of OP clinicians employed at hospitals is to promote a systems-based method of health of the bones and to educate themselves, together with their patients, about assessment, diagnosis, treatment, and prevention of diseases. Medical outpatient groups coordinating care with hospitals are given a chance to implement the same systems-based institutional approach. Priorities from this standpoint include dedicating staff to certain important tasks and using benchmarking information and academic details to improve care quality. Coordinated care can also involve the implementation of evidence-based conduits of care and use of computerized reminders to facilitate the provision of timely treatment. Some groups can initiate specialized OP care centers or clinics and incorporate external hospital programs for OP management.[3]

Patients with OP, when broadly defined simply as low bone density, are treated fully or partially in outpatient settings. However, despite the high prevalence of OP, most hospitalized OP patients are unaware of the condition, which has therefore not been treated prior. Studies have revealed that more than 80 percent of elderly patients with recent or new fractures such as hip fracture often are not treated for OP in spite of the high likelihood that the fractures developed as a result of depleted bone mass and/or low bone density. There are numerous effective medications for OP and also a high risk of future fractures for both women and men, and preparation is necessary for hospitals to (a) help manage inpatients just in case the fractures resurface, (b) make adjustments to daily life to avoid further bone degeneration, and (c) avert fractures at early stages of OP disease progression.[4]

Some OP experts also suggest that for the long-term care of hospital residents, particularly those at increased risk of falls and OP, under normal circumstances do not usually get the recommended assessments related to risk factors of decreased bone mass density. This, in turn, can lead to undertreatment, which is becoming more commonplace. Inadequate attention to the detection, diagnosis, and treatment of OP usually results in the need for hospital-based care nurses, who may be working in long-term care facilities, to handle issues pertaining to OP treatment. The goal here is that all OP patients are correctly diagnosed with the condition and treated successfully.[5]

Especially in high-risk and hospitalized patients, the bone health groups or teams, basically the healthcare professional teams dealing with fractures, have a key duty to boost patient education about OP. They also ensure that patients who may be susceptible are evaluated for the risk of OP and related fracture vulnerability, thereby enhancing the provision of preventive services and therapeutic treatment. Again, the nurses are vital to ensuring the success of these interdisciplinary efforts: They are responsible for addressing OP care by doing assessments for OP, general bone health, and risk factors associated with bone degeneration.[6]

All told, hospitals employ the nurses who play a key role in caring for patients with OP or at risk of developing it, provide educational services pertaining to knowledge regarding OP, and promote behavior change to help reduce the aggravation of the condition. Osteoporosis care also involves specific educational matters which, when nonexistent, would lead to decreased bone lifespan and fractures associated with OP. This applies to adolescents/young adults and also to older people who may be at high risk of OP. Treatment strategies, whether nonpharmacologic or pharmacologic, are always discussed by health professionals. Some of the nonpharmacological avenues of OP management include:

- Education of patients (along with family members who take care of them) on reducing risks of falls that might lead to fractures
- Providing nursing care to the patients and reducing associated complications, and
- Promoting medication adherence and lifestyle modification.

Seminars organized at hospitals augment health education, particularly with the sharing of experiences by patients and caregivers concerning treatment and management. Classes in the hospital also discourage OP patients from smoking and excessively drinking alcohol. During these meetings, all manner of questions can be answered and the latest OP research can be discussed. Not only is OP covered, but also other medical conditions known to threaten human life. Interestingly, seminars offered by hospitals can sometimes get complex in terms of attendance, as patients and caregivers may have differing schedules. The nurses in the wards often help with what is normally the responsibility of orderlies and nutritionists: positioning the patients properly, serving them the required diet, and educating them about which types of foods to avoid. The hospital's medical officers—MDs or staff physicians—prescribe the medications and, when necessary, surgeons operate on OP patients suffering from fractures. Bones cannot always be repaired when the issue concerns a lower limb. In certain cases, the only alternative is amputation. This process is done in the OR by surgeons, while hospital-based anesthetists aid in the process by administering the needed numbing or sleeping agent. Psychologists in healthcare institutions also play a significant role, counseling the patients in dealing with the difficulties associated with OP that may be hard to accept.[8]

When patients undergo testing for BMD, they can get an explanation for their health concerns and also take the necessary measures to try to avoid the risks for developing OP. This is significant because this testing can only be accomplished in hospital facilities. Analyses require the use of heavy machinery housed in hospitals because outpatient clinics often lack both budget and space for these instruments. The results of these tests can be interpreted either in the outpatient setting or at the hospital. Once conclusive results are available, hospital nurses are responsible for monitoring the array of medications, especially the ones affecting OP complications previously detected per imaging studies and bone densitometry.[9]

QUALITY OF HOSPITAL CARE AND TREATMENT OUTCOMES

Hospitals and physical rehabilitation centers sometimes move beyond their traditional role in simply treating bone-related indicators and also develop strategies to improve the overall health of the bones and joints. In hospitals, lifestyle mitigation involves increasing calcium and vitamin D intake as well as introducing exercises appropriate to the patient's age group. There is no cure for OP, but with proper treatment the bones are strengthened and protected. Skilled nursing care homes implement measures to prevent fractures and falls, including educating patients about the importance of consuming enough vitamin D and calcium and activities crafting a stronger bone frame, such as mild weightlifting. Health insurers often assess OP care and also monitor the performance of providers through a process known as utilization review.[10]

Hospitals and large health maintenance organizations (HMOs) should engage in programs for quality improvement and also implement performance and pay initiatives. Government agencies and the public health system are responsible for promoting clinical flowsheet–based bone care. This includes encouraging nurses and physical therapists to provide as much education to patients as possible. For higher-quality care, for-profit hospital sectors ensures their workers are well trained for their jobs—such as those involving direct treatment of OP—and are involved in the promotion of bone health measures and activities. This sector is also critical when it comes to reinforcing the existing link between community healthcare organizations and nonprofit hospitals to identify patients who might be at risk of fractures so that their care can be managed. As a result, people's bones become more durable and less bone breakage occurs within a given population as time progresses.[11]

A system-based approach can also be facilitated by large clinical-care institutions through research, purchasing policies, and education programs organized for the benefit of the population. Health providers such as OP doctors see to it that their patients are managed well and recommend specialists to their patients as needed. Some general physicians are extremely knowledgeable about OP, and some institutions have such doctors on staff; if not, patients with severe cases are referred to outside specialists. This is often how specialists who deal only with bone-related diseases get involved. The department dealing with bones that wear or have decreased mass may differ from one hospital institution to another; for example, in some facilities the department dealing with endocrinology and metabolic disease of the bones can actually treat OP sufferers, but in others, the branch responsible for orthopedics or gynecology will try to untangle the problem. Some hospitals have a separate program for OP or have a relationship with a health clinic for women that also manages OP cases.[12]

Treatment outcomes are directly related to the quality of care being offered in the inpatient setting, so those whose bones deteriorate quickly are often treated by qualified personnel in settings such as assisted living facilities with an unusually high number of OP sufferers. These institutions hire competent doctors and nurses qualified to provide medical services needed by OP patients, but they do this by way of careful coordination with a hospital. Medical imaging departments in hospitals treating OP should be well equipped with the necessary instruments to examine the body from head to toe, paying particular attention to the suspected areas of reduced bone mass and starting the measures to help them heal or to avoid fracture. Patients are often put on prescription drugs when OP is observed; physicians prescribe the medications depending on the extent of the bone density loss and ensure that these remedies are correct after assessing the patient. They also take a history of the use of other drugs that could be responsible for bone reduction or are contraindicated with OP medications. Some bones get too brittle with excessive loss in mass and often these cannot be rejoined in case of fractures; in these cases, suitable measures must be taken to facilitate surgery, such as encouragement from a psychologist if the client refuses to undergo certain procedures in inpatient surroundings.[13]

The role of hospitals in increasing knowledge about OP among both female and male patients is key because this is where the most critical cases wind up. Some elderly patients might find it difficult to address their condition. This group is at risk of developing OP but may not be aware of what is happening, so education is a key function of hospitalists (full-time hospital-based physicians), as they are responsible for monitoring the patients around the clock. Caregivers should note that a significant number of senior citizens have reduced knowledge on one's susceptibility to bone disorders in general.[14]

Patients undergoing chemotherapeutic treatments and who have other musculoskeletal disorders are also at increased risk in the hospital setting. Luckily, osteoporosis medications tend to counter the risk of fractures. In the hospitals, patients are educated about these matters to increase their understanding of the causal factors of OP along with possible complications that may arise and how they can be controlled. Studies have revealed data indicating that the unemployed and those with lower incomes have increased risk of developing OP, and physicians should know how to assist those who are in need of financial assistance.[15]

The activities and behaviors of OP sufferers also have a significant impact on the development of bone conditions. Individuals involved in vigorous activities can develop reduced bone mass over time but be unaware of the situation, resulting in spontaneous bone defects or fractures. Hospitals always monitor OP patients known to be current or former athletes for fitness before clearing them to resume such activities.[16]

Vitamin K supplementation may reduce the risk of fractures in postmenopausal women. Vitamin K, which helps reduce the process of bone loss and is vital for bone health, is not manufactured in the body, meaning it must be included in the diet. Sources of vitamin K include leafy green vegetables like kale, spinach, watercress, and lettuce. Potassium is crucial for slowing down age-related degeneration of bone mineral density. Other vitamins and mineral salts that are important are magnesium, vitamin C, and vitamin K2. Magnesium plays a vital role in treating and preventing OP, working with calcium to strengthen bones. When all said and done, hospital nutrition departments are more multidisciplinary than even the largest of outpatient private practices. They provide nutritional supplements when needed, of course.[17]

Under normal circumstances, caregivers tailor educational interventions using language that can be understood, based on cultural perspectives and possibly specific ethnic groups, as they educate OP patients on matters surrounding bone disorders. These healthcare professionals often explain the meaning and consequences of the disease along with some of the factors known to elevate the chances of stumbling and having fractures. These caregivers have an understanding of the depth and breadth of the disease and how to treat it. Nurses are adept at the administrative procedures that are accurate and correct concerning treatment, because an overdose will cause complications while an "under-dosage" may render the medication ineffective.[18] Medication provision involves many factors that have to be considered, including that (1) they are administered with water, (2) they are offered right before meals, (3) they must not be included with other medications, and (4) the OP patient should be upright and maintain such a position for 30 minutes.[19]

Most successful OP interventions in hospitals are associated with numerous methodologies: for example, OP self-management combined with education. Other strategies can also be incorporated, such as devising the health beliefs of the patients and their attitudes on OP added to the recommendations offered by the doctors, which include the medications as a common instruction from the physicians. The health beliefs are key for the adoption and maintenance of healthy behaviors related to OP treatment and prevention. Self-efficacy and patient expectations of the outcomes play a critical role in adherence to dietary behaviors, prescribed exercises, and medications by adults with OP. All of this is indicative of an inpatient setting.[20]

Being diagnosed with OP can be discouraging, as patients know they have debilitated bones that can easily break or are brittle enough to cause severe fractures. Using prescription drugs has some effect. Intravenous (IV) medications given in hospitals may cause headache, fever, and muscle pain that can last for several days. Taking these medications for years and years, however, is often counterproductive because that increases the likelihood of breaking specific bones, such as the thigh bone. Osteoporosis patients hospitalized with broken bones also have an increased risk of developing bedsores because their mobility is limited; simply lying on the hospital bed can lead to more problems if the caregiver is negligent. Lengthy stretches of hospitalization may also lead to poor performance of physical activities that may cause pain, and long-term patients who are still of working age may find their careers suffer as a result, causing financial difficulties. If the patient is the family breadwinner, the family social and economic dynamics are affected, as are the patient's children. The condition also often makes patients feel sick mentally, not just physically, hampering their quality of life. For the elderly, sometimes life expectancy is shortened even when they receive superior treatment at top hospitals. Males affected with OP have reduced life expectancy, and because of their comparatively heavier frames and higher daily energy usage, they tend to die earlier. In most cases, women do not face death from OP complications (from a pathology standpoint), but it is possible.[21]

As OP reduces bone density, the likelihood that surgery will be required to sublimate the underlying issue, especially in the extremities, is rather high. The stress resulting from surgical intervention can reduce the quality of life overall. It can also lower patient morale and outlook on life because once OP is established, it cannot be eliminated, only managed and treated to maintain bone strength. Prescription drugs used to treat the disease may also cause complications such as heartburn and stomach difficulties. As OP increases the risk for fractures, patients live knowing that at any time their bones may break, since the rate of bone loss may be so severe that even medications cannot reverse the situation.

Managing the emotional health of patients suffering from bone conditions helps maintain good visceral health, however. One thing patients can do to maintain emotional health is join support groups, which help patients realize they are not alone in their struggle. In these groups, people with OP discuss and give hope about their condition, particularly in terms of how the hospital has helped them through assorted medical hurdles. Emotions are associated with depression, but preventative education also helps get rid of the latter because then those affected can engage in physical activities and avoid tobacco intake as well as alcohol consumption.[22]

ANALYSIS

Hospital facilities have the equipment, financial resources, and human resources to aid in managing OP. The standard of care patients receive for their condition—including the quality of patient education and the professionalism of the healthcare teams—determine the outcomes of treatment and care. Inpatients suffering from OP face many challenges, such as the adverse effects of intense hospital drugs, long cycles of hospitalization, and the risk of getting fractures concomitant with reduction of individual quality of life.[23]

II
CLINICAL PRESENTMENT

5

Risk Factors and Causes of Osteoporosis

THERE ARE MYRIAD RISK FACTORS RESPONSIBLE FOR OP, SOME OF which society as a whole cannot eliminate completely. Therefore, at the very least, knowledge of these factors is necessary for diagnosis and development of treatment for patients. Clinical factors vary from population to population, but all these factors cause fracture formation. All the risk factors discussed here lower the optimal bone mass or accelerate bone loss. These features include familial anamnesis, genetics, hormone levels, food quality, physical activity, life habits, and overall health. Risk factors are classified as either variable or invariable.[1]

INVARIABLE RISK FACTORS

Invariable risk factors, which are either inborn or inherited from our parents, cannot be controlled. This array of factors includes age, sex, genetics, physical constitution, and race.

Differences in bone physiology between the sexes begin to reflect in puberty. In boys in puberty, androgens (the major sex hormones in males) and growth hormone lead to an increase in external bone size and in the size of the medullas duct as well as the thickening of a bone called the cortical bone. Androgens encourage the proliferation of osteoblasts (bone cells that build up bone), inhibit osteoclasts (bone cells that degenerate bone), and stimulate the synthesis of bone marrow proteins responsible for creating solid bone mass.[2] Females are medically different from males as far as OP and many other facets of healthcare are concerned. Estrogen (the major sex hormone in females) inhibits periosteal (outer frames of bone) growth, resulting in narrowing of the medullas duct. Because of this, the bones of men after puberty are larger than the bones of women.[3]

In 30 percent of males, OP is a consequence of another illness (e.g., anorexia nervosa, hypogonadism, rheumatoid arthritis), the use of medications (e.g., glucocorticoids, anticonvulsants), or the consumption of alcohol and tobacco (secondary OP). In men younger than age 60, if there are no other causes of the disease, the diagnosis of idiopathic OP is applied. Involutional OP (regressive alterations to bone mass from aging) occurs in men over the age of 60 as a result of an involution process similar to that seen with postmenopausal OP in women. Healthy men have about 25 percent more bone mass than women of the same age. The bone marrow in males has significantly more bone mass than in women.[4]

In postmenopausal women, the process of degradation and bone buildup is unbalanced. Everyone gradually loses bone mass over the years, irrespective of health status, as the relationship between decomposition and bone building in the organism is disturbed. When the degradation process becomes faster than the bone-building process, OP develops. About half of all women will eventually suffer from some form of OP as a result of the lack of estrogen after menopause. Because symptoms of OP may not develop until bone loss is extensive, it is important for women at risk for OP to undergo regular bone testing.[5]

Substantial Variation in Fracture Risk among Different Age Groups

The treatments vary for OP that presents during childhood and adolescence. As part of the natural bone-building process, new bone is added in haste while the old bone is removed. This means that during the phases of childhood, adolescence, and young adulthood, bone becomes heavier, larger, and denser, respectively. At the age of 30, reaching peak bone mass is a significant goal. Factors affecting bone remodeling are:

- Stress to the skeleton via hard workouts and physical activities
- Hormonal influences
- Weightlifting exercises[6]

Osteoporosis is a major health issue in pediatrics. Childhood OP is generally a consequence of genetic bone abnormality or an underlying medical condition or its treatment. Immobility, pubertal delay and other hormonal disturbances, and malnutrition and low body weight can contribute to the development of OP. Physical activity builds bone mass in youth and maintains it in adulthood. When a person is immobile, osteoblasts are unable to work as well. Weightlessness and immobility can likewise result in bone loss. For example, astronauts are exposed to the microgravity of space and experience significant bone loss. After returning to Earth, their movement is difficult because bones have weakened.[7]

Studies in immobile people have shown drastic bone loss. During the time spent in bed, there is an increased loss of calcium and phosphorus in the urine and often higher blood calcium levels. When a person recovers mobility afterward, many of these levels will return to normal and bone loss will stop. Immobility for more than six months is a risk factor for OP. Physical activity during growth increases bone mass in children. Teens should get at least an hour of physical activity every day and adults should get a minimum of 30 minutes for optimal bone health.[8]

In the absence of physical pressure, the bones and joints may not bear weight for a while, increasing the chance of bone loss. Bone strength and mass might be lost due to immobilization and paralysis. However, primary OP can be considered common among all age groups, while secondary OP is less prevalent but still important. Secondary OP is characterized by a bone loss in larger amounts than that expected from an unaffected individual of same gender, race, and age. Common causes of this are excessive alcohol consumption, inadequate intake of vitamin D and calcium, limited to sun exposure, and sedentary lifestyle.[9]

Age is an important risk factor that should serve in determining whether to refer patients for medical testing in hopes of an early diagnosis of OP. In this way, with appropriate therapy one would prevent possible breaks. The body of the woman in menopause is changing as hormone production in the ovaries, especially estrogen, has been reduced. The formation of hormones in the ovaries begins to weaken after about age 40, and even earlier in some women. The reduced production of estrogen in menopause, known to be a substantial risk factor of OP, results in a change in bone metabolism. However, postmenopausal OP can be prevented and treated. The best prevention and treatment method in postmenopausal women is hormone replacement therapy, which may also be used to stabilize bone. Although men have a lower risk for OP than women, they do still develop it, generally later in life. Because men tend to be older when they get OP, the complications from broken bones—most often hip, spine, and wrist bones—can be more serious for them.[10]

Primary OP is often called "idiopathic osteoporosis," meaning its cause is usually unknown. Idiopathic OP involves men under 70 years of age. Unlike idiopathic OP, causes of secondary OP are known; they may include medications, illness, or lifestyle. Some causes of secondary OP in men include glucocorticoid medications and other immunosuppressive drugs, hypogonadism, chronic obstructive pulmonary disease and asthma, cystic fibrosis, gastrointestinal disease, hyperparathyroidism, immobilization, and lifestyle elements covered later in this chapter.

*Hypo*gonadism (not to be confused with *hyper*gonadism) is a low level of sex hormones. Testosterone levels generally decrease as men age, but a sudden decrease can cause problems. Glucocorticoids and many other factors may cause this sudden drop. Studies have shown that hypogonadism can be a cause of OP in the male population. Men with hypogonadism have low estrogen levels, which can cause bone loss. Other risk factors for OP in men include kidney, bowel, and lung diseases; certain drugs; race; and smoking and heavy alcohol consumption.[11]

Long-term use of some medications may increase the risk of OP because some medications can accelerate bone loss. Corticosteroids cause OP and fractures in a high percentage of patients. The effect of corticosteroids on BMD reduction has been examined in depth, and studies have shown the connection between corticosteroids and BMD reduction. Steroid medications, in the broader sense, have major effects on the metabolism of calcium and vitamin D, impacting bone health. This can lead to bone loss, OP, and broken bones. Postmenopausal women who take steroid medications for longer than six months have the greatest risk of bone loss. Almost one in three postmenopausal women who routinely take steroid medications will have a spine fracture, and an OP patient on steroids is more than twice as likely to have a spine fracture than an OP patient not taking steroids.[12]

Breast cancer has a special relationship with bone health because of the hormone drugs often used to treat it. Estrogen is important for maintaining bone strength in women, so breast cancer treatments that act against estrogen can lead to the weakening of the bones. Corticosteroid reduces the concentration of estrogen and testosterone in the blood and may slow down the building-up of bone or reduce bone mass. Glucocorticoids modify osteoblast cell differentiation, number, and function. The most significant effect of glucocorticoids in bone is the inhibition of bone formation, which is brought on by a decrease in the number of osteoblasts.[13]

One of the conundrums is that in many of the underlying diseases where corticosteroids are used, bone loss may already be present. In patients with long-standing rheumatoid arthritis (RA) who had not been treated with corticosteroids, there is significantly reduced BMD at both the lumbar spine and femoral neck regions of the body, generally speaking. People with RA of less than six months' duration were found to have a BMD that was normal, but over a 12-month of follow-up period, the rate of bone deterioration was greater than that of control subjects with early bone loss. Patients with uncontrolled RA also lose more bone compared with those with well-controlled disease.[14]

People with inflammatory bowel disease (IBD) and those who have received organ transplants have a higher risk of developing OP compared to healthy groups. Inflammatory bowel disease includes Crohn's disease and ulcerative colitis, and some individuals with these conditions have lower than average bone density. In some patients, this takes the form of OP while in others, it is osteopenia (low bone density) or osteomalacia (softening of the bones). These two bone abnormalities occur more frequently in people with Crohn's disease than in those with ulcerative colitis and are more common in women than in men. Many with Crohn's have OP at the age when they should be at peak bone density: age 20 for women and age 30 for men. Thousands, if not millions, of people around the world suffer from IBD. The prevalence of osteopenia associated with it varies significantly depending on the study population and location.[15]

Low BMI in inflammatory bowel disease may be an additional factor leading to the development of OP. People with IBD are often treated with glucocorticoids such as prednisone or cortisone to reduce the inflammation caused by their disease.

Over time, these drugs interfere with the development and maintenance of healthy bones. Bone loss increases with the amount
and length of glucocorticoid therapy. Severe inflammation of the
small bowel or surgical removal of components of the small bowel
can lead to difficulty absorbing calcium and vitamin D, posing
another cause for concern.[16]

People with type 1 diabetes typically have low bone density.
Insulin may promote bone growth and strength, but in type 1
diabetes it is deficient. Type 1 diabetes usually occurs at a young
age, when bone mass is still increasing. It is possible that patients
with this form of metabolic sugar imbalance achieve lower peak
bone mass, increasing the risk of developing OP later in life.
Some people with type 1 diabetes also have celiac disease, another
condition associated with reduced bone mass. It is also possible
that cytokines, substances produced by various cells in the body,
function in the development of both type 1 diabetes and OP.[17]

LIFESTYLE IN CONNECTION TO OP

Scientists have unearthed the connection between lifestyle and
OP. Healthy bones need dark leafy greens, whole grains, fruits,
nuts, and calcium-rich foods. Diets heavy in processed foods,
refined sugars, and high-sodium intake are a disaster for bone
health. Lifestyle is a variable risk factor, which can be changed if
people alter their lifestyle, reducing the risk of illness by reducing
or eliminating bad eating habits. Healthy activities and habits
include exercising regularly; eating a balanced, nutritious diet;
getting adequate sleep and relaxation; abstaining from smoking
and nonessential drugs; and moderating the intake of alcohol.[18]

Enjoying a healthy, balanced diet with a variety of foods and
an adequate intake of calcium is a vital step to building and maintaining strong, healthy bones. Calcium is essential for building
and maintaining bone. Eating a diet containing enough calcium
is an important way to preserve bone density. Just about all of

the body's calcium is found in the bones, but every day, calcium is excreted from the body via sweat and urine. This loss requires sufficient calcium intake on a daily basis, because if there is not enough calcium in the blood, the body will take calcium from bones. If insufficient amounts of calcium are consumed, the para-thyroid glands begin to produce parathyroid hormone (PTH) in much larger amounts, leading to changes in metabolism rate. The best way to get the recommended level of calcium intake is to try to consume a diet rich in calcium.[19]

Excessive alcohol use is a serious health risk, and that risk includes effects on bones. Excessive alcohol use, often during the adolescent and young adult years, can dramatically affect bone health and increase the risk of developing OP later in life. Put simply, heavy drinking disturbs the balance of calcium in the body. Alcohol interferes with the production of vitamin D, which is essential for calcium absorption. Overconsumption of alcoholic beverages can also cause hormone deficiencies. In men, hormone deficiency results in lower production of osteoblasts (the cells that stimulate bone formation). In women, it results in irregular menstrual cycles, which reduces estrogen levels. Alcohol also affects the level of cortisol in the body. Cortisol increases bone breakdown and decreases bone formation, and in people with alcoholism, cortisol levels may be elevated. People with alcoholism also tend to stumble more frequently than others, resulting in a higher risk of broken bones.[20]

In a similar vein, there is evidence that smoking has an impact on bone health. Research suggests that smokers begin to lose their bone mass more rapidly than nonsmokers, once symptoms of OP are in full swing, increasing their risk of fractures. Nicotine and other toxic substances in cigarettes cause many changes in the body, including the bones. They reduce the blood supply to bones and slow down the production of osteoblasts. Tobacco con-sumption affects the absorption of calcium and leads to a rapid breakdown of estrogen in the body. In women, smoking may cause early menopause. Smoking also increases the risk of fractures and makes bone healing more difficult. If a person smokes for only a few years, the risk of fracture is reduced.[21]

PHYSICAL ACTIVITY AND IMMOBILITY

Physical activity always has beneficial effects on patients suffering from OP. Physical activity contributes to a healthy energy balance and increases muscle mass and bone mass. Exercise also has an added benefit on bone density of postmenopausal women. People who exercise experience less bone loss. Swimming and water exercise are not weight-bearing exercises. Hence, they are great forms of activity for senior OP patients. Walking at high intensity improves bone health, muscle strength, fitness, and balance. Elderly individuals with OP should avoid abdominal sit-ups, forceful movement, strenuous golf swings, and other exercises with a forceful twisting motion outside of supervision of a professional caregiver or health professional. People with OP should have 45 minutes to one hour of aerobic activity two to three times per week and resistance training two to three times per week. To reduce the chances of a bone fracture, it is necessary to continue this exercise routine in the long term.[22]

PHYSICAL AND MENTAL STRESS LEADS TO OP

Many studies have investigated the effects of physical stress on bone. Physical stress is a mechanical load; depending on the kind and exercise intensity, it can be deleterious. Intense sports activity may lead to OP. Physical activity causes changes in bone metabolism that can be direct, via mechanical force. or indirect, via hormones. The mechanical force interferes with the processes of bone remodeling. Factors that directly affect the bone include cell deformation caused by direct force over the bone cell, the pressure increase caused by dynamic force, and the increase of the interstitial fluid flow. Intense sports activity does not protect women against bone loss in menopause, but the moderate physical activity has beneficial effects on the bone tissue and in OP prevention.[23]

Organisms are exposed to various stressful stimuli that affect physiological processes. Stress, mental and physical, leads to a disturbance of the balance of the organism, and in humans, this imbalance can cause the diminishing of calcium in bones. Bodies respond to stress by producing the hormone cortisol, and increasing cortisol levels in the body. Calcium also helps neutralize the pH of the cortisol, helping restore the body's "acid versus alkaline" state to neutral. The osteoblasts are reduced, and that, in turn, inhibits the ability of the bones to regenerate. In fact, bones are constantly being leached of calcium, resulting in porous bones, brittle bones, and OP.[24]

Clinical evidence suggests that persistent psychological stress can lead indirectly to OP. One study compared more than 2,000 depression patients with more than 20,000 nondepressed individuals to determine the relationship between depression and skeletal health. The depression patients showed lower bone mineral density. Both osteoporosis and depression are about three times more common in women than in men. Women are more sensitive to both physical and mental stress and more vulnerable to depression-related low bone mass. Several studies of the relation between OP and depression in men indicated that bone loss over 24 months was greater in depressed men than in control subjects and that bone mass in depressed men is lower than bone mass in nondepressed men. The hip BMD of these subjects was lower than in nondepressed subjects.[25]

CULTURAL AND ENVIRONMENTAL RISK FACTORS FOR OP

Ethnicity and race influence the prevalence of OP. Asian women tend to be slenderer on average and have less bone mass than heavy women and are at greater risk for osteoporotic bone fractures. Calcium is essential for bone building and people should consume it for maintaining a healthy skeleton, and many Asian diets are low in calcium. Asian American women are more prone than women of other races to lactose intolerance and have trouble digesting milk products. They may avoid dairy items, the primary source of calcium in the diet, increasing their chance of developing OP.[26]

Many African American women consume less than the RDA of calcium. African Americans are also prone to lactose intolerance. Hispanic females have a greater chance of developing diabetes, which may increase their risk for OP. Caucasians and Asians, however, have the highest risk of developing OP. It is estimated that 15 percent of Caucasians over the age of 50 and as high as 70 percent over the age of 80 have OP. The frequency is higher among Asians and in the Australian population than the European and North American population. African Americans boast the lowest risk, and American Indians have a moderate risk. People of different races have different BMD. Studies have found that African Americans have higher BMD than Caucasians. This difference is the consequence of genetic differences.[27]

Ethnic and race variability is much lower in vertebral fractures worldwide. For example, for Caucasian women the prevalence of vertebral fractures is 70 percent; for Mexican women, 55 percent; for Japanese women, 68 percent; and for African American women, 50 percent. Caucasian men tend to have higher hip fracture rates than Asian and African American men, but ethnic and race variability is much lower for men. Ethnicity and race also influence where the fracture associated with OP occurs.[28]

Although the risk of hip fracture is more profound in Caucasian women than in African American women, mortality after hip fracture is higher in African Americans. The reasons for this have not been fully established, but it could be older age at time of fracture, greater comorbidity, or disparities in healthcare received. Caucasian women suffering from OP have screenings for BMD a lot more often than African American women of the same cohort.[29]

ANALYSIS

Physical activity is important for muscles, not only for bones. Smoking and drinking too much alcohol and other ill-advised habits are not good for the physical integrity of bones. Approximately 12 million Americans over age 50 have OP, which leads many experts to conclude that age is a contributing factor of OP. Postmenopausal Caucasian and Asian women are at the highest risk. Half of all women over age 50 and a quarter of men above 50 will break a bone due to OP. This bone-density related condition also causes broken hips in men, although not as often as in women.[30]

6

Pathology of Osteoporosis

PATHOLOGY IS THE STUDY OF THE NATURE OF DISEASE AND ESPE-
cially of the functional and structural changes that are produced
by it. One cannot start from the top downward, but instead must
move from the bottom upward, meaning they have to first understand the disease process and its signs before drawing a conclusion. Doctors must first understand the process of a disease, how
it reproduces and spreads, and how it can be differentiated from
other, similar diseases before determining a diagnosis, in this case,
OP. It is easy to confuse OP with other bone diseases such as
osteoarthritis, Paget's disease of bone, osteopenia, hyperparathyroidism, and arthritis, among others. So, then, pathology of OP
will be regarded as the study of the distinctive features and characteristics that set it apart from all other bone disorders.[1]

PATHOLOGY AS A STUDY OF SIGNS AND SYMPTOMS RATHER THAN DIAGNOSIS

As one grows old, the bones thin and get flat, which makes them
susceptible to breakage. Fractures are very likely if OP has set in
because that means that bones have become very weak. In younger

people, the bones are in a continuous state of regeneration. younger people make new bone at a faster rate than their bodies break down the old bone, leading to increased bone mass. In the elderly, bone mass is diminished because the rate of formation of new bones is reduced. The lower bone mass leads to a decreased bone density, which is the more distinctive sign of OP. It is caused by the body's failure to produce new bone at the same rate as the old bone wears out.[2]

Different diseases often present similar signs and symptoms, and doctors must be keen on ruling out the similar ones that lead to an inaccurate conclusion. This process of elimination can be done with laboratory testing, in the case of OP, for calcium, vitamin D, and other substances. Radiography is done to detect the presence or absence of swelling, flattening and widening of intervertebral discs, and other signs. DXA scans are very accurate in determining the porosity of bones. All these tests and procedures are done so the pathology of the patient's OP is understood and minimizing the chances of error during diagnosis and treatment.[3]

Another critical aspect to keep in mind concerning the pathology of OP is the fact that it's a "silent" disease that might be present in the body for a long time before a fracture occurs. The sure way to prevent fractures is by trying to avoid falling or accidents, but this is challenging because fractures in OP patients are sometimes caused by minor falls in the course of reaching for or bumping into something.[4]

Rheumatoid arthritis also hastens the disease progression of OP, since the bones are already weak due to a reduction in synovial fluid. This increases friction at the joints, leading to pain in the hips and wrists. It is said that OP tends to run in families. As a result, older adults from families with a history of OP should be on the lookout. Another group at higher risk is adults who take medications known to increase the chances of getting OP. These medications include injectable contraceptives, cancer drugs such as tamoxifen, and steroids.[5]

It should be noted that children and teens can also suffer from juvenile OP, which generally occurs between the ages of eight and 14 during growth spurts. It is more severe than OP occuring later in life because it presents when the bone structures are still in the formation process. Juvenile OP can either be secondary and idiopathic. Secondary OP is caused by an underlying medical disorder of joints (such as arthritis), leukemia, kidney disease, and malabsorption syndromes, among other conditions. Idiopathic juvenile OP has no known cause. Notably, fractures in juvenile OP are most prevalent in the ankles, feet, and legs, while pain is usually localized in the hips, knees, lower back, and feet.[6]

Usually, the first symptom of OP is fracture, since the bones are already fragile. Fractures are common because in people with OP, it doesn't take a serious accident, but rather mild to moderate trauma, to cause them. Patients find that OP fractures might be caused, for instance, by a fall from just below standing height, the mild impact caused by falling, tripping, or hitting an object. Usually, patients and caregivers will notice that the objects that cause fractures in OP patients are so light they would not have ordinarily produced a fracture. So when a rather mild accident causes a fracture, that indicates the patient's bones are worn out and very weak because of OP.[7]

Osteoporosis fractures are most prevalent around the wrist, hips, and spine. People over age 50 experiencing these fractures should talk to their physician about bone loss tests and screening. The outcome of these tests will determine the treatment options that should be discussed between the doctor and the patient. It has been found that very few women experiencing fragility fractures knew they had OP beforehand, and most people are prompted by a fragility fracture to ask their doctor about their bone health. Relatively few individuals begin follow-up management intended to prevent another fracture.[8]

How do patients know whether their fracture is fragility related? This is a valid question because fractures in OP patients are not always apparent. In a fragility-related fracture, the injured area swells and becomes painful immediately after an impact or fall that wouldn't ordinarily cause serious injury. The fracture can also cause the affected area to look out of alignment. Sometimes, patients feel pain—say, in the back—but are unable to attach it to a single incident. It is important to note that sometimes back pain can be the result of a vertebral fracture. Vertebrae are bones lining the spine, one on top of the other. They connect to form a passage that protects the spine. As these bones become weak, they tend to flatten out, narrowing the passage. This puts the spine at a high risk of irreversible damage. In the case of vertebral fracture, the pain can last up to six weeks as the bones heal. Whatever case it may be, patients should discuss injury management with their doctor.[9]

Another sign of OP is physical changes such as a change in posture or a loss of height. A stoop, sometimes called a dowager's hump, may also be an indication of OP. Osteoporosis may cause the bones of the spine to break without experiencing any pain, causing the spine, over time, to curve inward and the affected person to develop a stoop or become shorter. Doctors are usually advised to regularly measure patients' height, especially in those over age 50, to monitor any changes that generally arise due to age. If a change in height of more than 2 inches or a spine curvature is noted, these symptoms should be noted; it means that OP is affecting the patient's vertebrae and putting the spine in danger. Patients who notice this stoop, should consult their physician and discuss ways to increase calcium levels in the body to correct it.[10]

Height loss is also among the presenting pathologies of OP. This could be caused by vertebral fractures and poor posture. However, poor posture does not necessarily indicate bone loss; it can also be caused by weakening of muscles surrounding the spine. Bones and muscles work in synchrony, which means they will also lose and gain strength in sync. When the bones of the spine thin and become longer, the vertebrae can easily break. These breaks may be painful but are sometimes not painful at all. When many of these bones break, the spine curves inward, causing a stoop. In the absence of obvious pain, people may not know their vertebrae are breaking and therefore may not seek medical assistance or take precautions against further damage.[11]

Another sign of OP is high levels of alkaline phosphates or serum calcium on a blood test. Also, a -2.5 or less BMD T-score indicates OP. Another early sign of OP is vitamin D deficiency. The central role of vitamin D is to make bones strong and denser, so in patients lacking this mineral, the bones become weak and easily susceptible to fractures. Consequently, the low vitamin D level worsens the situation. Calcium, a mineral, is essential in the body to fight against OP. This is because calcium aids the body in taking up vitamin D. So they work concurrently in keeping the bones healthy. Tests for BMD and vitamin and mineral deficiency are all done in the laboratory or by a professional, further explaining why OP is referred to as a silent disease—no one is going to have their blood taken and tested without any apparent ailment. [12]

Other signs of OP include muscle or joint aches. This could be because as we age, synovial fluid is reduced, causing friction in the joints. This explains why rheumatoid arthritis is a risk factor for developing OP. Also, in people with OP the bones are already weak and less dense, which means they can't hold onto the muscles firmly, leading to muscle pain in case of strenuous work. People with OP may also experience difficulty standing upright from a chair without using their arms to help.[13]

Caution must be taken not to conclude that all muscle and joint aches are signs of OP. It should be noted that in people over age 50, pains and aches are very common and may be caused by different things. This is because as we age, the body becomes weaker due to a reduction in the production of new cells. In younger people, the body produces new cells at the same rate it loses them. But over time, this process slows and the rate of production of new cells doesn't match the rate of loss. This leads to a lot of different ailments.[14]

If bone loss is not severe, then just weight exercises and lifestyle changes may be recommended along with treatment for the associated pain. Calcium and vitamin D tablets or supplements may also be prescribed. In women who have just reached menopause, estrogen replacement may be given, either transdermal or orally. However, estrogen replacement should be taken with care since it has been associated with certain cancers, coronary heart disease, vaginal bleeding, and strokes. These risks can be reduced with proper dosages and combinations of drugs.[15]

RARE SIGNS AND SYMPTOMS OF OP

Receding gums indicate weakness in bones. Bone loss is directly related to dental and oral health because 99 percent of the total calcium in the body is found in teeth and bones. It has been found out that bone loss in the mouth and jaw could indicate the same loss of bone in other parts of the body. If the bones in the jaw are deteriorating, the gums will follow the same trend and recede. Therefore, it is always advisable when brushing their teeth, people should note any changes in the gum line. Also, it has been found out that there is a connection between BMD and tooth loss. This is why postmenopausal women with OP are more likely than women with normal BMD to have tooth loss. People with receding gums also often have difficulty fitting their dentures because the BMD of the jawbone decreases with age.[16]

The primary causes of brittle fingernails are nutrition and hormonal changes. The unstable estrogen levels in menopausal women dramatically affects the strength of their nails, making them brittle. Besides causing frail fingernails, it also causes dry skin and thinning of the hair. Postmenopausal women with brittle fingernails, dry skin, and thin hair should visit their doctor to rule out OP. On a positive note, patients diagnosed with OP and started on treatment in its early stages have been reported to experience fingernail resilience. Hence, the issue of brittle fingernails is manageable if the underlying cause is treated early enough.[17]

Usually, patients diagnosed with OP are put on specific programs and the results are evident within months of starting the treatment. Note that weak nails could also be caused by nutritional deficiency—for instance, lack of calcium, folic acid, and vitamin C—so it is essential to maintain a balanced diet. Nails that easily split, chip, curl, or break are all characteristics of brittle nails. Also, discoloration of ridges and nail dryness could indicate nutritional deficiency associated with OP.[18]

Another rare sign of OP is weak grip strength. Everyone has opened a tightly sealed jar of spaghetti sauce at one point in their life. When people notice that the jars they used to open with ease have now become more difficult, the actual problem could be their bones. It has been found that grip strength is directly related to bone density. This means that the lower the bone density, the weaker the grip strength. In the same vein, studies have found out that decreased grip strength is associated with an increase in the risk of vertebral fracture because people with low grip strength have similarly low BMD measurements in the hip and spine. The good news is that this can be corrected by doing weight-bearing exercises. Consistent exercise of both the dominant and nondominant hands ultimately increases the grip strength.[19]

It is common to hear people say that old age is associated with pain. However, muscle aches should not be taken lightly, because they may signal inadequacy in vitamin D which is a crucial bone builder. Leg cramps that happen mostly at night could also signify low levels of magnesium, calcium, and potassium in the blood. If this condition is not resolved by taking supplements of those minerals, excessive bone loss may occur that might be irreversible.[20]

This spine or backbone curve is called kyphosis. With the continuous breaking of the bones of the spine, the curve gets more pronounced and is often called a dowager's hump. In some people, this curve can cause constant pain around the area, which is intensified when the muscles and ligaments of the back are stretched and strained as the spine continues to curve. When the nerves are pinched it becomes even more painful. Some spine fractures are not painful and usually resolve on their own. People who experience spine fractures that do not cause pain may not know they have a fracture until it is found on an X-ray. Severe kyphosis reduces space for internal organs like the stomach, heart, lungs, and others. This causes the abdomen to push forward, making breathing and eating difficult. As a result, patients with severe kyphosis may lack necessary nutrients because they are not eating enough, leading to other diseases associated with nutrient deficiency. Also, when breathing is difficult, the blood doesn't get enough oxygen, and that means the whole body lacks it. The lack of oxygen in the bloodstream can lead to the death of body cells and general body weakness due to decreased metabolism.[21]

ANALYSIS

Osteoporosis is a bone disease caused mainly by lack of vitamin D, calcium deficiency, and estrogen hormone imbalance. It can also be caused by other underlying medical conditions. Osteoporosis is common in old age, although it can also affect children and teens. Early signs and symptoms of OP include receding gums, weak grip strength, and weak and brittle fingernails. Later signs and symptoms include fractures from a fall, loss of height, stooped posture (dowager's hump), and neck and back pain.[22]

7

Genetics of Osteoporosis

ALL BIOLOGICAL SPECIES HAVE VARIOUS SIMILARITIES AND DIF-
ferences. For instance, humans have various common traits that
define the species as humans. Some of these traits include having
a spinal cord and a backbone, which categorize humans as mam-
mals. Humans further have traits that define us as primates that
stand upright on two limbs and have short body hair, small teeth,
a jutting chin, distinct lips, a flat face, and a prominent nose. All
these traits differentiate humans from other primates such as
chimpanzees. As biological organisms, people tend to inherit
these traits from their parents, but the inherited traits vary from
one person to another. The inheritance of these characteristics is
defined by genetics.[1]

INTRODUCTORY GENETICS OF OP

Genetics refers to the reception of common traits by living things
from previous generations. The genes of an organism contain its
DNA, the chemical instructions for the operations and construc-
tion of the organism. DNA is found in the genes of all living
things. Genes are also hereditary, and there's a region on the

chromosomes that leads the way for characteristics notable in an offspring. In this way, parents pass their characteristics on to their children, determining the appearance and the personality traits of the child. It was Charles Darwin who first came up with the theory of evolution, but this theory was brought to completion by Gregor Mendel, who pioneered the field of genetics. This was important to our understanding of how evolution takes place. Through his experiment on peas, Mendel discovered that it is a mixing of various factors, and not a blending of characteristics, that leads to heredity. The modern field of population genetics emerges from a combination of the current knowledge of genetics and Darwin's evolution theory.[2]

Apart from general characteristics, those traits that lead to variations in health are also inherited. Some of these traits include predisposition to Alzheimer's disease, mental depression, chemical dependence, diabetes, high blood pressure, and OP. The traits can be inherited culturally or biologically; for example, fluency in one's native language is a result of cultural inheritance, while the color of one's eyes is a result of biological inheritance. In terms of health, environmental factors and biological characteristics combine to influence traits, so that an individual's weight, for example, is a result of heredity as well as eating habits and physical activity.[3]

How Genetics Plays a Part in Musculoskeletal Disorders in General

In some cases, people suffer from degenerative musculoskeletal conditions that are mostly influenced by environmental factors. The pathogenesis and etiology of such conditions can be understood by studying the vulnerable genes that partially lead to them, but further studies are required in order to come up with improved treatment and diagnostic methods pertaining to these disorders. Musculoskeletal disorders common in adults include developmental dysplasia of the hip (DDH), degenerative disc disease (DDD), and osteoarthritis (OA) of the knee joint and hip. Studies conducted on these conditions have found various candidate genes as well as overlap between the genetic sources of these conditions. At a level of genome-wide significance, only a few genes have been identified and associated with these conditions. More research is required to identify these genes in order to come up with long-lasting remedy to these disorders.[4]

Due to the significant advances in the study of genetics that have been seen in recent decades, several genetic alterations can now be easily detected. These advances have also led to an increased understanding of the pathogenesis of and predisposition to musculoskeletal disorders. Despite this improved comprehension of these disorders, however, significant steps toward their treatment have not been made. While much of this recently acquired knowledge is aimed at aiding the diagnosis and the treatment of musculoskeletal disorders as well as better patient counseling, several discoveries have been made concerning the genes responsible for osteogenesis disorders, skeletal dysplasia, and various other Mendelian conditions.[5]

Projects are aimed at identifying the genes responsible for conditions like DDH, DDD, and OA. Researchers looks at complex developmental patterns on an ongoing basis. Several life-threatening complications and disabilities are associated with most of these musculoskeletal disorders, which generally affect the elderly and consequently tend to overburden the healthcare system. Many of these conditions are polygenic, meaning that both environmental and genetic factors are involved. In the development of new treatments, the pathogenesis and etiology rely mostly on the identification of the involved susceptible genes.[6]

The Future for Genetic Studies in Musculoskeletal Disorders

Much research has been conducted on the genes involved in musculoskeletal disorders; however, only a few genes have been discovered to be definitively associated with conditions like DDD, DDH, and OA. This is the result of numerous factors, including the heterogeneous nature of the disease and small sample sizes obtained from previous studies, and is also subject to various environmental and genetic factors depending on the affected areas. Currently, detailed sequencing methods are preferred for use over the genome-wide association (GWA) approach because it is a more cost-effective method of identifying candidate genes in musculoskeletal conditions. Patients suffering from extreme prosthetic joint infection (PJI) are an example of life-threatening end phenotype. In the absence of all excluding criteria, interest is in identifying the variance in DNA caused by genetic susceptibility leading to PJI. This approach is relevant in identifying the susceptible genes that result in PJI and various other musculoskeletal disorders.[7]

A variety of approaches are required to come up with more valid information in future. It is critical to making use of data from diverse, large-scale multiethnic genome-wide association studies (GWAS) to help in interethnic assessments, which are possible through global cooperative efforts. It is expected that future orthopedic surgeons as well as other healthcare professionals will have enough information related to genetics to aid them in managing musculoskeletal conditions and advising patients suffering from them. This knowledge is extremely important in understanding the etiology of these conditions. An understanding of genetics is also important in developing therapies and diagnosis in order to provide better medical care to the affected population.[8]

How Genetics and Heredity Play a Role in OP

The most serious skeletal disorder of older people is OP. The condition leads to physical disorientation of the bones and low bone mass, which increases the risk of bone fracture. This condition is becoming a global health problem. Recent statistics indicate that 30 percent of postmenopausal European and American women, along with hundreds of millions of people from other parts of the world, are suffering from this condition, which underscores the importance of coming up with a cure. Between 15 and 30 percent of males and 40 percent of females with OP experience a fragility fracture. Understanding the genes responsible for the development of and predisposition to this condition is fundamental for the development of innovative therapies and preventive measures for OP.[9]

Based on the guidelines of the International Osteoporosis Foundation (IOF), there are two classes of OP risk factors. The first class is fixed risks, which are invariable and innate; the second is variable risks, which are modifiable and largely subject to habits and nutrition. It is understood in the scientific community that this condition is very complex and that it arises from the interaction of environmental and genetic factors that impact bone metabolism and fracture risk. Research shows that variability in BMD as a result of genetic factors is at 60 to 85 percent. This effect becomes more prevalent with age.[10]

There also seems to be a genomic component of the fragility risk factor. A number of epidemiological studies have indicated that heredity seems to be a factors in fracture risk. However, more research indicates that fracture heritability is not influenced by BMD and that it is subject to various other factors, such as the risk of falling, bone resorption, and the shape of the bones. The impact of heredity, however, decreases with age as the effect of environmental factors kicks in. Various other factors that have been found to exercise control over genetic factors include the markers for bone turnover and the geometry of the femoral neck.[11]

The turnover of the bones is highly regulated by various genes with some exercising more control than the others. The complexity of the skeletal structure involves various candidate genes for suspected OP. Candidate genes for bone metabolism are continuing to be discovered. Some of these genes include those that regulate calcium and bone metabolism as well as those that regulate the proteins in the bone cell molecular pathway. The situation is made more complex by the interaction of gene-environment and gene-gene factors. A similar osteoporotic genotype can result from diverse environmental and genetic factors, making it possible to be genetically at risk of developing OP. Conversely, some individuals with no such genetic predisposition may become osteoporotic later in life as a result of nongenetic factors.[12]

A study to identify the candidate genes has revealed BMD-associated gene alterations and fragility fracture risk. However, the results obtained are somewhat conflicting as a result of linkage disequilibrium (the opposite of genetic linkage), gene-gene interactions, the absence of standard methods of genotyping, confounding factors, age, gender, ethnicity, inadequate sampling of the population, and gene-environmental interactions, among other factors. Various studies, as well as retrospective meta-analyses, are essential.[13]

OSTEOPOROSIS AND CARDIOVASCULAR DISEASES

Over the years, several studies have identified cardiovascular diseases (CVDs) and OP as independent diseases that arise as a result of age. However, recent studies have confirmed that the two diseases are actually related and that they have some common physiopathological mechanisms. The idea that the two diseases may be related raises the question of the involvement of genes in both cases. Various other studies have indicated that CVDs and bone loss as a result of age have some common etiologies. These studies have also indicated that women have a higher genetic predisposition to experiencing a hip bone fracture as a result of these conditions.[14]

Calcification is known to cover up to 90 percent of atherosclerosis fatty plaques. It has been discovered that calcium plays a primary role in the progression and development of arteriosclerosis as well as the mineralization of bones because vascular calcification can be affected by the functions of the regulatory factors for bone cells. The atherosclerosis and vascular calcification are a result of a protein called osteoprotegerin (OPG) that also functions as a regulator for the activation of the osteoclast. This factor might be the cause of calcification of the artery walls. Several other factors also contribute to vascular calcification and alteration of bone mineralization. Some of these factors include lack of physical activity, smoking, high fat intake, dyslipidemia, oxidative stress, chronic inflammation, estrogen deficiency, and low calcium and vitamin D intake. Most elderly people have a deficiency of calcium and vitamin D, which is known to cause excessive bone calcium mobilization. This can lead to the calcification of arteries and other vessels.[15]

Osteoprotegerin decrease is also caused by a deficiency of estrogen in the body. The OPG deficiency occurs due to the risk of high bone calcium mobilization as well as atherosclerosis plaque calcification. Estrogen deficiency also leads to lower production of nitric acid, which regulates bone microcirculation endothelial function and also osteoblast function. Low levels of HDL cholesterol and elevation of LDL cholesterol are said to play a role in atherosclerosis; they are also said to be one of the causes of vertebral fractures as well as low BMD. Alteration of the metabolism of lipids plays a role in atherosclerosis as well as the remodeling of bones. To some extent, this explains how OP and atherosclerosis coexist in patients suffering from dyslipidemia.[16]

ANALYSIS

Osteoporosis is one of the most complex musculoskeletal conditions ever known. It is associated with a number of factors, such as heredity and environmental conditions. From a genetics standpoint, this issue seems to mostly affect elderly people, with post-menopausal women being twice as likely than men to be affected. A number of treatments for this condition have been identified, but there's no treatment available as the absolute cure for OP.[17]

8

Mental Aspects

DEPRESSION IS ONE OF THE MOST COMMON AND WELL-KNOWN mental illnesses, and it often affects those suffering from OP. Good emotional health is a major issue in people with OP because a lack of it encourages the feeling of fragility and old age. Bones keep regenerating so that people can keep up with physical activities. However, patients with OP may think that vigorous physical activity can worsen things, although this is a myth. This mistaken belief can trigger a depressive state in the mind, causing even more problems in the future. Unhealthy lifestyle practices—including smoking, very low body mass index (BMI), alcohol, and sleep disturbances and deprivation—are the bridge connecting OP and depression.[1]

THE LINK

Research shows that there is an often-overlooked link found between OP and depression that causes as much as a 50 percent increase in fractures in the United States. Other studies have shown that those with depression have a higher rate of decrease in BMD compared to OP sufferers without depression.[2]

APPROACHES TO OP DEPRESSION

The good news is that emotional health and depression are indeed manageable. Aside from maintaining good health, there are several approaches people with OP can take to manage their emotional health, and these proven and effective approaches can be used to reduce the possibility of bone fractures. The use of the self-administered Patient Health Questionnaire-9 (PHQ-9) is one approach that aids in finding the best treatment of emotional health and depression management in individual patients. Using the system-based approach, experts are able to identify three significant phases in managing depression: (1) the initiation phase, (2) continuation phase, and (3) the maintenance or follow-up phase.[3]

- In the initiation phase, the goal is to minimize the symptoms of depression. This phase follows known treatments for depression, including those for depression associated with OP. Generally, this phase promotes support groups and counseling, use of antidepressants, and psychotherapy.
- The continuation phase involves six months of medication using antidepressants for the first and subsequent episodes of depression, for long-term remediation is the ultimate goal.
- The goal of the maintenance/follow-up phase is preventing relapse of emotional health problems or depression in people with OP. To achieve the best outcomes, patients should follow-up within two to four weeks after starting therapy, and continue to do so on an ongoing basis.

MEDICATIONS FOR DEPRESSION

Although doctors do use other approaches to treat depression in OP, pharmacologic therapy is the most popular. Pharmacological therapy is an approach that primarily uses drugs or antidepressants as the main remedy to manage mental health. The medications used may include selective serotonin reuptake inhibitors (SSRIs), tricyclic antidepressants (TCAs), serotonin/norepinephrine reuptake inhibitors (SNRIs), St. John's wort, atypical antidepressants, monoamine oxidase inhibitors (MAOIs), and serotonin-dopamine activity modulators (SDAMs).[4]

Most people with depression associated with OP are given SSRIs as their main treatment for emotional health problems. This is because the low possibility of toxicity in overdose often makes it the best treatment not only for adults but also for adolescents and children. Commonly prescribed SSRIs include escitalopram (Lexapro), citalopram (Celexa), paroxetine (Paxil), fluoxetine (Prozac), vilazodone (Viibryd), fluvoxamine (Luvox), vortioxetine (Brintellix), and sertraline (Zoloft).[5]

Though their effectiveness has been known for years, compared to SSRIs, TCAs have high toxicity in overdose, so they are not often prescribed to treat depression in people diagnosed with OP. Some TCAs include doxepin (Sinequan), amitriptyline (Elavil), desipramine (Norpramin), clomipramine (Anafranil), imipramine (Tofranil), trimipramine (Surmontil), protriptyline (Vivactil), and nortriptyline (Pamelor). SNRIs are generally the first-line agents in treating OP patients with depression, pain syndromes, and fatigue. Commonly prescribed SNRIs include duloxetine (Cymbalta), venlafaxine (Effexor), levomilnacipran (Fetzima), and desvenlafaxine (Pristiq).[6]

St. John's wort (also known as *Hypericum perforatum*) is a different medical approach to depression in people with OP, as it is an over-the-counter herbal remedy that is commonly used in Europe. Those seeking first-line treatment of mild to moderate emotional health problems, including depressive symptoms, St. John's Wort is a great option.[7]

Individuals with OP who also suffer from anxiety disorders often use MAOIs because of their potency. However, these medications must be accompanied by a low-tyramine diet to prevent the risk of adverse effects such as weight gain, insomnia, and sexual dysfunction, among others. Furthermore, these medications increase the risk of hypertensive crisis, so those taking them should carefully follow the prescribed dosage and diet. Some MAOIs include tranylcypromine (Parnate), phenelzine (Nardil), isocarboxazid (Marplan), and selegiline (Emsam).[8]

Aripiprazole (Abilify) and brexpiprazole (Rexulti) are the most common SDAMs. The former is known to treat bipolar mania, schizophrenia, and Tourette disorder, while the latter is best used for major depressive disorder (MDD) and those individuals with OP who complain of other mental health.[9]

OP AND MOOD SWINGS

The correlation between OP and depression has been theorized alongside the idea that experiencing fractures in OP may be a considerable factor leading to depression. However, there is only a weak support for this theory. Further research has shown that anxiety, mood swings, stress, and other emotional health problems are a factor in causing the decline of bone density, thus increasing the risk of fractures when not treated with antidepressants.[10]

In modern times, it is expected that MDD, like mood swings and anxiety, will be second only to hypertension as the leading cause of disability worldwide. This is an important note for patients and caregivers alike. Presently, it is still unclear whether OP causes depression or depression causes OP and the significant loss of bone density leading to fractures. Everyday activities at home and at work are affected in people with chronic pain, often resulting in depressive symptoms such as mood swings and stress. Because chronic pain is impairing the function of the body in everyday life, people suffering from it find it difficult to perform tasks involved with daily living, reducing their self-esteem and well-being and diminishing their quality of life.[11]

Research suggests that mood changes, anxiety, and depression have a profound impact on physical health, especially in women. More than 1,000 Finnish women between the ages of 60 and 70 were studied. The study concluded that women who were satisfied with their lives had higher BMD, while those who were unsatisfied had lower BMD.[12]

Another research study was performed to explore the correlation between bone density and mood changes in men. In 2015, men from Australia between the ages of 24 and 98 were studied for an initial assessment using the data from the Geelong Osteoporosis Study. This study concluded that MDD can cause a decrease in BMD.[13]

Even in the early stages of MDD, low BMD is pervasive. Mood swings, anxiety, stress, depression, and other forms of MDD result in OP because of two significant factors: lifestyle and hormonal influences. Even minor changes in lifestyle are believed to play a major role in both physical and psychological health. Unhealthy lifestyle practices make people more susceptible to decreased BMD, making them prone to fractures and falls. Poor diet, lack of exercise, low vitamin D, physical inactivity, low calcium intake, excessive alcohol intake, tobacco use, and low nutrient intake are among the factors that can worsen mental health.[14]

Although OP is a skeletal disorder, bone remodeling is controlled by hormones released by the hypothalamus. This pertains to the frequent changes encountered in the hormonal pathways causing concurrent problems of both bone and brain. This is common in situations involving inflammatory cytokines as well as the decrease in levels of estrogen and progesterone. While mild mood swings are considered a minor form of mental disorder, they are often attributable to depression and should be treated promptly. Treating mood swings and other forms of depressive symptoms that cause chronic pain can help patients protect against the loss of BMD.[15]

Experts emphasize, however, that the use of antidepressants is also related to lower BMD, particularly in men. Long-term use of antidepressants in the treatment of depression should be carefully monitored and avoided if possible, especially if the patient has already been diagnosed with OP. The best way to manage mood swings and other depressive symptoms associated with OP is without the use of fervid drugs. Though there are alternative therapies available, it is still better for the doctor to discuss approaches with the OP patient. Effective ways to manage mood swings include:

- Avoiding the most common triggers for mood swings, such as stress, caffeine, lack of sleep, erratic schedules, certain medications, and substance abuse, among others.

- Learning effective coping strategies.

- Exercising regularly. This is a great basic approach to managing mood swings because it prompts the body to release endorphins that help improve mood and control stress levels. Endorphins are hormones that interact with the brain and the entire nervous system; they have an analgesic effect, resulting in the reduction of pain.

- Getting enough sleep. This can help improve mood, improve appetite, and increase energy level.

- Tracking moods and maintaining a good schedule. This helps people learn to regulate and facilitate the highs and lows in mood and energy.

- Getting proper nutrition. Maintaining good diet avoids overconsumption of harmful substances such as caffeine and sugar and helps regulate mood swings.[16]

Therapy is another great approach to dealing with mood swings. It also helps people learn to handle the triggers of stress that may arise during day-to-day activities. Psychotherapy and cognitive behavioral therapy (CBT) are the best ways to treat mood swings and disorders and to track patterns and behavior. Psychotherapy is a great treatment option for mood swings and disorders, including the depressive symptoms associated with OP. Otherwise known as talk therapy, it helps manage the symptoms of emotional and mental health problems. This approach works for children, teens, and adults. Psychotherapy may be conducted in one-on-one sessions with the patient or it may include the patient's family, a couple, or a group. Sessions generally last between 30 minutes and one hour and can be short term or long term, depending upon the complexity of issues. This approach is often used together with medication such as antidepressants to treat hormonal imbalances and is often associated with a healthy lifestyle.[17]

In CBT, mood swings and depression in OP patients are treated using a combination of cognitive and behavioral theories. CBT mainly focuses on the actions and behaviors of the patient. The therapist helps the patient to recognize unhealthy patterns and negative beliefs—such as exaggerated circumstances, black-and-white thinking patterns, emotion-based snap conclusions, negative bias, worst-case scenarios, and overlooking the positive—and devise strategies to overcome them.[18]

Another treatment for mood swings and other depressive symptoms, including those connected to OP, that has been found to be effective over the years is acupuncture. Acupuncture is believed to help equalize the subtle energies in the body and increase the production of dopamine, norepinephrine, and endorphins, resulting in a positive mood. Acupuncture is believed to release serotonin, a neurotransmitter in the brain that manages the moods, aggression, anger, sleep, and other forms of discomfort. The best thing with this approach is that it does not come with harmful side effects while rebalancing the hormones in the brain, stabilizing fluctuations in hormone levels, and removing the energy blockages.[19]

APPROACHING OP-RELATED ATTENTION LAPSES

Attention lapses are one cause of fractures in people with OP. This problem is most common in the elderly, but it can also appear in children. In the worst-case scenario, people who experience attention lapses—especially the elderly—sadly might be labeled as inconsiderate or lazy. Attention lapses during the daily routine are unpredictable and may cause larger problems for seniors with OP, resulting in fractures and accidents. These lapses in attention may also trigger factors that cause depression in people with OP. Commonly known as absent-mindedness, these lapses generally result in minor problems, for example, the inability to recall where to find something. However, there are also some major or life-threatening forms of attention lapses which make people with OP most prone to mental health issues.[20]

Studies show that even the relatively small, everyday attention lapses can cause difficulty for OP patients. Using a cognitive failures questionnaire (CFQ) provided to patients of clinics by clinical research companies, researchers are able to determine the correlation between attention lapse and depression. Fortunately, attention lapses are treatable, and the most common treatment is the use of a stimulant, which has been found to effectively reduce attention lapses in children, adults, and elders. When investigating the effects of stimulant medication among children with attention deficit hyperactivity disorder (ADHD), scientists were able to determine mental response time. Among the medicated children, the variability of response time was reduced compared to those who were unmedicated. Attention lapses in people with OP may be related to ADD symptoms. Although the use of stimulants for elderly patients with attention lapses has not been tested, it is likely that outcomes would be similar.

Furthermore, unlike in the measures of memory performance, attention lapses and memory failures are uncorrelated with age, which explains why the use of mental stimulants in people with OP is also expected to be effective.[21]

Many seniors experience emotional problems, such as thoughts of loneliness, sadness, worry, and boredom, especially if they are coping with the loss of a spouse, other relatives, and friends. Unhealthy diet, emotional problems, mood swings, stress, anxiety, and depression cause a person to be more forgetful and produce attention lapses. Emotions always play a major role throughout elderly life. This makes emotional health a vital consideration, especially if they are also dealing with OP symptoms. Treatment with stimulant medications, along with exercise, healthy diet, and happy surroundings, can help stabilize their emotions and lessen attention lapses.[22]

OSTEOPOROSIS AND MEMORY

Just like OP, problems with memory are common in the elderly. These memory lapses maintain a constant change with age, especially when societal burdens and emotional problems surface. In the worst-case scenario, studies have shown that people with OP are more likely to develop Alzheimer's disease (AD). Seniors diagnosed with AD more often experience OP-related falls and fractures compared to other elderly people.[23]

Studies have revealed a correlation between dementia and OP. In one case-control comparison, patients with and without OP were examined. This study found that around 20 percent of women with OP and 16.4 percent of control subjects were determined to have dementia. Similar results were found for male subjects: Roughly 20 percent of those with OP and 15 percent of those without were diagnosed with dementia.[24]

Studies indicate a strong correlation between the two in both men and women of the elderly community. Between 10 and 15 percent of women with cognitive impairment, including memory lapses, will develop AD in their future years. Common causes of memory lapses and loss include factors such as medications, tobacco, alcohol, drug use, sleep deprivation, nutritional deficiency, stroke, head injury, sleep deprivation, and dementia. There are also secondary factors of memory loss such as tuberculosis, HIV, and syphilis, all which affect the part or whole brain.[25]

The cause of memory lapses in an individual patient is a crucial factor in treating them, and in many cases they are reversible. For instance, the OP drug known as raloxifene (Evista) is a selective estrogen receptor modulator (SERM) drug that is FDA approved for use in the prevention and treatment of OP in women. Evista, which is also taken by postmenopausal women to reduce the risk of breast cancer, mimics estrogen in the bone, reducing the occurrence of fractures in bone in women with OP. The drug may also be used to treat memory problems in postmenopausal and elderly women. Evidence shows that it can lower the risk of mild cognitive impairment, including memory lapses and loss, up to 33 percent after three years.[26]

Two other types of medications used for the treatment of Alzheimer's disease, reasoning problems, confusion, memory loss, and other cognitive symptoms in patients (with or without OP) are the memantine (Namenda) and cholinesterase inhibitors (Razadyne, Aricept, and Exelon).[27]

Cholinesterase inhibitors are drugs to treat language, thinking, judgment, and memory problems in early to moderate stages. It is well-tolerated as it delays or slows worsening of symptoms of memory lapses and prevention of acetylcholine breakdown. Galantamine (Razadyne), donepezil (Aricept), and rivastigmine (Exelon) are the most commonly prescribed cholinesterase inhibitors. For OP sufferers in moderate to severe stages of memory lapses, confusion, and other cognitive problems, it is advisable to take memantine (Namenda) combined with donepezil (Namzaric). Memantine is effective in regulating glutamate and improves mental ability to perform daily activities with few side effects.[28]

ANALYSIS

Solving the disambiguation between mental health and OP is an important step in finding a cure to bone degeneration, whatever the triggers of the depression. Though there are no concrete answers to the question of whether depression is caused by OP or OP is caused by depression, the best defense against both is to live a healthy lifestyle. Antidepressants, therapies, and alternative medicines play a major role in the treatment of mental health issues, but doctors should still be on the lookout for unwarranted self-medication.[29]

9

How Osteoporosis Affects Everyday Life

SINCE OP IS A DISEASE OF THE BONES, IT AFFECTS ALL THE activities of life. The actions affected may range from reflexes such as coughing and sneezing to a bit of strenuous work like lifting and intense farm work, among others. Even simple activities such as walking and reaching for something become tricky in the advanced stages of OP. Daily routines of life such as going to the toilet, showering, bending to pick something up from the floor, or straightening out the bedsheets may become nearly impossible. Almost like an enigma, it is difficult to know when there is pain involved or not, and yet the daily routines of life cannot get done. That explains the reason why OP is referred by many as a silent disease—because for many, it is not diagnosed until it is too late.[1]

ACTIVITIES AFFECTED BY OP INSIDE THE HOME

Osteoporosis patients are often afraid to do any chores for fear of sustaining fractures or experiencing pain. As a result, they must ask for help to do most of the work they want to be done.

This can make them feel helpless, vulnerable, and burdensome to their families. This can result in depression, which, as discussed in chapter 8, can lead to other health ailments. Osteoporosis patients have nervous breakdowns because they can't do their favorite recreational activities such as swimming, biking, and dancing, among others. Just about every activity they undertake warrants a call for help on their part. As a result, they feel they have lost their independence. Caretakers and family members should always hope the best for OP patients and reassure them in a positive manner.[2]

People who have retired from the workforce often strive to keep themselves busy doing activities they love, which keep them active and give them pleasure. These activities may include gardening, taking care of pets, spending time and playing with grandkids, and the like. Elderly OP patients might find it hard to do these activities because they don't want to hurt themselves or sustain fractures. Caregivers find that individuals with OP rest often, perhaps balancing their weight against a large garden tool or resting on a stool, to avoid the onset of pain. This way they can continue doing the activities they love, but with caution. People in the advanced stages of OP, however, are unable to do heavy activities such as mowing the lawn, digging, or lifting flowerpots, so they must rely on friends and family or employ paid help.[3]

Elderly OP patients often need help getting dressed. This can be uncomfortable, especially when undergarments are involved. A married patient being helped to dress by a partner is one thing, but it can feel awkward for older adults who need to be helped by a nonfamily caregiver or even a younger family member. It feels like their privacy is being infringed. Everyone needs a bit of privacy, but, unfortunately, OP patients might not always have this. The act of pulling a pair of pants up, for example, requires energy, which exerts pressure on already fragile bones. As a result, people with OP might sustain more fractures, making them even more vulnerable. To avoid this, OP patients require help when dressing, ideally by a friendly and approachable caregiver. Diagnosed

OP patients should not wear high-heels or other uncomfortable shoes; it is advisable that they wear shoes that allow a firm grip on the ground, hence avoiding slipping or falls. The shoes also must fit well, as painful feet may affect overall stability.[4]

The use of a washing machine makes caring for clothes easier for OP patients, although they may need help with items that must be washed by hand. Bending to get to the level of a washbasin puts pressure on an already brittle spine, and weak knees might not be able to support the weight of the body. A basin can be put on a high stool so that washing doesn't require excessive bending, or a family member or caregiver can also help wash clothes. When the patient is a premenopausal woman going through her period, an empathetic close family member can wash these items for her to avoid causing embarrassment and discomfort.[5]

Cooking can be dangerous for OP patients because there is a high risk of accident. Activities such as putting a roast in the oven may create pressure on the already weak spine, making it more prone to fractures. Barbecuing is very dangerous as there is a burn risk in the event of a fall. Generally, OP patients should keep far away from fire, as the chances of an accident are so high and may lead to severe burns. Even just merely tripping might lead to a dreadful accident as their bones are already weak and cannot always adequately support their weight. Moreover, most OP patients have already sustained fractures and often either walk with a limp or bend forward constantly. Such persons should not be around fireplaces or do any complicated cooking. Simple cooking can be done with the help of a caregiver or family member. Osteoporosis patients can use a grabber tool to bring hard-to-reach items closer in the kitchen. This avoids overstretching and possibly kitchen falls. Any spills should be cleaned immediately to prevent slipping, which could result in a fall that causes fracture.[6]

There is an increased chance of accidents while bathing because of slippery surfaces. Protruding water taps and showers should be covered, or better still, avoided completely. A long stool should be used in the bath to eliminate overstretching. Shower organizers should be installed to arrange shampoo, soaps, and other bath products in one position to eliminate unnecessary bending. The bathroom should be amply lighted to avoid fumbling around in the dark. For those OP patients who find it difficult to move into and out of the bathtub, a bath seat should be provided so they don't keep attempting to move around in the tub.[7]

A handheld shower that can be used while seated should be installed so that OP patients don't have to stand for long stretches of time under the showerhead. Likewise, floormats with rubber backings should be put on the floor to provide a firm ground and minimize the chance of an accident. Osteoporosis patients often find it hard to move from a sitting to a standing position, making it difficult to use the toilet. This can be made easier by installing a toilet seat riser or a frame with a mounted armrest. If the bathroom walls are tiled, bars should be fixed into the wall studs for OP patients to hold for support.[8]

Mothers with OP who have young children are advised not to lift their young ones from the floor. Instead, they should sit on a firm chair with the baby on their lap. This prevents compression fractures in the spine, which can be caused by bending over too much. For children who need to be carried, are crying, or otherwise need attention, the mother should ask for assistance. Any action done in haste by an OP patient may lead to more fractures and pain. Osteoporosis patients should never be left at home alone with young children, as this can lead to home accidents. Children are always spilling drinks, throwing objects, generally making the household more prone to accidents. There should always be another alert adult in the house to clean up spills and pick up the littered objects in and around the house.[9]

Osteoporosis patients are advised not to carry and lift heavy objects, whether the item is on their shoulders or being lifted from the floor. Objects of a reasonable weight may be safely lifted off the floor by bending at the knees and carried at chest level (never over the head), and OP patients should not overreach for items high up in a cupboard or on a shelf. These precautions will avoid putting strain on the spine, which can lead to compression fractures.[10]

Most OP patients have to make adjustments to their homes to minimize the risk of accidents. They might have stairs installed with sideways handles that they can hold as they move up and down the steps and extra lighting to help them see clearly where they are going to avoid tripping or missing a step. Care must be taken not to leave any clutter on the stairway, as this can also lead to accidents. Uneven staircases must always be repaired to minimize falls. Scatter rugs should not be in the house, since they can slide and cause falls. If the house must have rugs, they should have a firm backing, and if possible, they should stick to the floor. In addition, there should be no protruding furniture in the house. Every piece of furniture must be placed well to reduce the hazards of mishaps. Stray furniture should be put away.[11]

OP patients should use canes or walkers to increase their stability as they walk around the house. Physicians suggest the use of walkers because they provide more support and stability. Walkers and canes distribute body weight over a wide area, providing firm support. As a result, they give a sense of independence and reduce the fear of falling. Canes and walkers come in different forms and fittings, so a physiotherapist should be consulted for advice on which one to buy, specifically fitted for the patient. Chairs should be fitted with a seat lift, a device put under a seat that pushes the sitter upward. This helps OP patients avoid exerting pressure on the chair as they get up, minimizing the chances of sustaining fractures.[12]

Medications and over-the-counter drugs should be taken with care. Some of these medications, especially antidepressants, can cause a drop in blood pressure, which can be very dangerous for OP patients as it may cause fainting. Sedatives can cause drowsiness, causing a loss of balance. When both these types of medications are being taken at once, OP patients are confined to the home, which means outdoor activities cannot be done. Even short walks outdoors can be very dangerous for OP patients after taking sedatives and antidepressants. Branded food supplements are bought over the counter or are prescribed by a physician in stronger doses. Many have the word *natural* written on them, but they can also lead to side effects such as drowsiness and dizziness. These can never be trusted entirely as they can lead to gait imbalances and falls. Products with these side effects should be avoided as much as possible to minimize the risk of accidents.[13]

ACTIVITIES AFFECTED BY OP OUTSIDE THE HOME

Driving a car is an activity that is immensely affected by OP. Driving requires the use of both legs and hands—and of course, the mind. Many osteoporosis patients cannot use their legs and hands to do strenuous work such as driving a car. Similarly, since their spine is already weak, they can't sit or bend for long periods of time. For OP patients who love driving and do so as a hobby or recreation, restrictions on their driving can be frustrating. Some people save up for years to buy the car of their dreams. Some people possess an especially strong love for vintage vehicles, which they want to enjoy after their retirement. Coincidentally, OP also sets in at about the same time, and they may find they have saved the money to buy a car that in the end they can't drive. This can drive them into depression (no pun intended). They can still enjoy the luxury of their car, however—with the help of a driver. The driver can either be a paid one or a family member.[14]

Icy surfaces must be approached with strong caution. Osteoporosis patients can attach ice grips on their shoe soles to aid in walking on ice, but they should always watch out for low-traction areas and avoid slipping. Icy surfaces are hazardous and pose a threat to anybody and therefore should not be taken lightly.

Anti-slip devices should not be trusted fully to prevent falls. Caution should be taken not to enter malls and stores with anti-slip devices attached, as they are slippery on indoor surfaces, especially tiled floors. Canes or walking sticks should have a sharp or rubber tip on the end that prevents slippage. This minimizes the risk of accidents while walking on ice. Outside balconies, staircases, and walkways should be kept clear of ice and snow to prevent slips and falls.[15]

People whose bones are weakened often find it hard to do their normal shopping routine. This is because it involves work such as lifting and picking heavy materials from the shelves and pushing shopping carts around, risking fractures and pain to already weak bones. From a psychological standpoint, it might be difficult to entrust another person to do the shopping; they might not pick the right color of cloth, the right brand of perfume, the right flavor of pastries, and so on. It even gets more difficult for people who are very particular with their shopping and would likely never be satisfied if another person did their shopping for them. For these people, when OP sets in and they can no longer do their own shopping, it feels such as a part of them has died. Therefore, such individuals need to be continuously reassured and taught measures of living positively with OP while learning alternative ways of shopping. These might include online shopping and home delivery, which allows them to select the items of their choice as though they were physically present in a store.[16]

As discussed earlier, exercise is a critical factor in the management of OP. Exercises should be tailored to avoid heavy straining. Weight-bearing exercises such as low-impact aerobics, yoga, walking, and muscle stretching exercises are very effective in keeping the body strong. These exercises stretch and beef up the bones in the legs, hips, and lower spine. In this way, mineral loss, especially calcium and vitamin D, is minimized. OP patients should consult a physiotherapist to determine what exercise regimen to undertake, as some may be dangerous to OP patients; for instance, OP patients cannot carry weights in the gym as they exert pressure on the already fragile bones, thereby increasing the risk of fracture.[17]

When OP patients go out to eat, they should ask for a comfortable seat that doesn't strain the back. When asking for a seat, there is no need to explain the medical reason; OP patients can just ask for a comfortable seat and eat the food they want.

Precautions should be taken if and when driving. When driving, OP patients need to watch out for the cars behind and to the side of them using the side and rearview mirrors. This reduces the risks of twisting and sudden turning that might break the already weakened bones of the arms. While riding in the car, OP patients should sit comfortably with a pillow behind their back for support. In case of sudden braking or hitting a bump, the pillow acts as a shock absorber, reducing the impact between the body and the car and minimizing the chance of breaking brittle bones. When entering or exiting a car, OP patients can swing their legs inward or outward while seated, facing the door. This avoids unnecessary turns and twists that can lead to fractures and pain.[18]

When using public transit, OP patients should carry a pillow or comfortably thick clothing to provide extra support. They should avoid traveling during peak hours, as they are too crowded and there is a greater risk of being knocked off balance. When it comes to OP, a slight fall or even staggering can easily cause fractures. When alighting a busy bus or train, one should wait for everyone else to get out and then exit last to avoid being squeezed by the many people alighting at the same time. Those who need help with this shouldn't hesitate to ask for it. This could be a helping hand for support to stand upright, extra light when the stairs are otherwise dark, or even assistance carrying luggage. People nearby do respond to calls for help, so no one should shy away from asking for it.[19]

Depending on the severity of the condition, newly diagnosed OP patients may still be working on a full-time or part-time basis.

They might feel generally strong and fit, despite being diagnosed with OP, and decide to keep working. In this case, then the office chair at the workplace must be fitted with extra pillows for comfort and to reduce the weight of the body onto the chair. Also, OP patients can take short walks periodically to reduce the time spent seated in one position. They can take the stairs instead of the elevator, being careful not to miss a step. This is a form of exercising that strengthens the leg bones. If they live close enough to their workplace, they can wake up early and walk to work instead of driving. If they live farther away, they can take a bus halfway and then walk the rest of the distance.[20]

Strenuous activities such as cycling, playing tennis, and golf should be done with care, if at all. They require forward bending (which exerts pressure on the spine), twisting, and bending at the waist. All these activities can lead to compression fractures in OP patients. Any exercise that requires forward bending or twisting forcefully at the waist are not recommended by doctors because they increase the chances of fractures. Examples of these include sit-ups and bending forward to touch the toes. In the same way, high-impact exercises such as jumping, jogging, and running should also be avoided. OP patients find it hard to do these activities because they exert force on already weakened bones. Rapid and jerky movements should be avoided altogether, and OP patients should instead opt for slow, gentle, controlled movements. However, those who generally feel strong and fit despite having OP can engage in higher-impact exercises. For those patients, slow, gentle workouts might be boring, so consulting a physiotherapist is a good idea depending on how determined the OP sufferer is.[21]

Analysis

Because OP is a disease that affects the bones, daily and routine household undertakings ranging from bathing, washing, cooking, lifting heavy objects off the floor, and even just reaching outward are affected. The way OP patients interact with their children and pets is also affected. Outdoor activities affected include driving, shopping, exercise, going to public places, as well as using public transport on a regular basis.[22]

III
Resolutions

Prevention

THERE'S A SAYING THAT "AN OUNCE OF PREVENTION IS BETTER than a pound of cure." This is true when discussing any medical condition, not just OP. Many different diseases cause death, and a majority of these deaths could have been avoided if a preventive care plan had been in place. Aside from improving the length and quality of people's lives, prevention can also reduce the significant economic burden associated with disease.[1]

THE IMPORTANCE OF PREVENTION

As the words themselves imply, preventive care is focused on keeping disease from occuring by maintaining good health and wellness. Before any symptoms of the sickness or illness in question are present, prevention stops the illness from happening in the first place. In terms of medical conditions, prevention might mean having a healthy lifestyle, good diet, regular exercise, and making all possible efforts to keep the body well. Aside from this, preventive care also extends to annual and routine examinations, laboratory tests, immunizations, and even counseling, all of which provide for a healthier lifestyle.[2]

Spotting a clinical problem before it worsens and becomes difficult to cure is the main goal and importance of preventive care. Instead of dealing with medications and the process of curing the disease or the condition, the main objective of preventive care is to keep patients from developing the condition. If the sickness is avoided or detected at an early stage, some of the possible negative outcomes might never arise. Osteoporosis patients can treat early signs using milder nonprescription medications, which are less expensive compared to their prescription versions. Postdiagnostic medications are always more expensive than preventive supplements. Aside from the cost, when caught early, many diseases can be nipped in the bud and full health restored quickly. Because of this, it is important to become educated about specific illnesses like OP and their symptoms as well as the treatments and what it takes to maintain good health overall.[3]

Once the preliminary stages of the illness are detected, it is critical for OP patients to visit their doctor on a regular schedule, either annually or possibly more often as the person ages, to stay healthy and keep symptoms from worsening. If detected early enough, a full cure is much more likely, which makes it less likely that serious complications will arise that involve debilitating symptoms or loss of life. This is one of the main goals of preventive care. Osteoporosis-related pain is another factor that preventive care helps tackle. When a preventive care plan is in place, the patient will not have to deal with the huge amount of pain that goes hand in hand with the symptoms of the illness. Without pain, OP patients can proceed with their regular daily schedules and go on with their lives. Whenever a certain condition like OP isn't detected early through preventive care, treatment could cause disruption in daily activities.[4]

Preventive care can also reduce overall medical expenses. Illnesses diagnosed in their later stages usually require a great deal of medical treatment to manage. Many of the required medications and procedures are very expensive. When preventive care is done and the disease is detected early, instead of going through a variety of medical procedures to treat OP, patients can instead do simple checkups and procedures aimed at thwarting the sickness instead of curing it. In extreme cases, some medical conditions occurring with OP may lead to severe financial loss due to the amount of treatment required and its cost.[5]

After treatment, individuals with OP might end up bankrupt because of the costs of the required medical procedures. By spending a fraction of those funds on preventive care and avoiding the actual illness, there is no financial loss at all, and instead the person's hard-earned money can be spent on vacations with the family or investments. The vast majority of elderly patients have chronic conditions that overwhelm their daily activities, or they are weighed down by medical diagnoses that ultimately raise their health insurance premiums. Learning about and practicing preventive healthcare, like maintaining the body and good health throughout the lifespan, is arguably the best method to prevent disease from materializing in the first place. If a specific illness is prevented, the aftereffects will be avoided, too. This is a critical advantage of preventive care. When patients are sick to the bone, all they ever think about is their illness. They lose hope and sight of what is in front of them. Some even let their condition take over their lives. When this happens, the consequences are felt by the OP patient and the family.[6]

Family members often have a hard time dealing with patients because of the effort it takes to make them feel like things are the same as they were before. This is one of the enormous impacts brought about by sickness or illness, whereas if the specific medical condition had been prevented and avoided, patients and their family members could just go on with their lives as normal. Simply put, disorders such as OP can cause debilitating illness and death among people who would have an excellent chance of surviving and living a full life if only the disease had been detected earlier. If early detection had been done through the process of preventive care, then the lives of these people would be a lot better. Aside from saving lives, preventive care also aims to prolong lives by helping people understand the need to focus on their health, especially as they age.[7]

HOW TO PREVENT OP

Osteoporosis patients as well as healthy individuals should follow a nutritious diet with adequate calcium intake. Since OP is a condition that weakens the bones, making them fragile and easily breakable, it is a given that to prevent it, people need to have enough calcium in their body from as early an age as possible. Parents should make sure that the food their children eat has enough calcium to help strengthen their bones and keep OP from developing in the future. Examples of foods high in calcium are milk, yogurt, sardines, beans, lentils, canned salmon, cheese, leafy green vegetables, whey protein, tofu, nuts, and bread. Many other foods are also rich in calcium; physicians can provide a more comprehensive list that can serve as the basis for a daily diet that prevents OP from developing. Adequate supply of vitamin D is also crucial to preventing OP. The main function of vitamin D in preventing OP is that it increases the intestinal absorption of calcium and other minerals. If the body is better able to absorb calcium properly, then the daily intake of calcium can also be adjusted to match an appropriate level. Even after an OP diagnosis, higher levels of calcium in the body can help strengthen the bones. Foods rich in vitamin D include fatty fish like tuna and salmon, orange juice, and dairy products.[8]

The following is a list of a few general ways to prevent sickness or illness. These are useful in the prevention of OP and other medical conditions.

- Eating a proper and balanced diet
- Getting regular exercise

- Visiting the doctor regularly
- Having regular visits from professional caregivers in the healthcare field[9]

These may seem like common sense, but starting with just these four tips have a great impact in preventing illness.

Now that both the meaning and importance of preventive care in general have been covered, it is time to discuss the advantages of prevention more specifically in connection with OP.[10]

Maintaining a bone-building diet is important for OP patients. In addition to including foods rich in calcium, a bone-building diet also involves staying away from those foods that can increase the risk of developing OP due to bone loss. Soft drinks have a damaging effect on BMD because they are high in refined sugar and simple carbohydrates, also known as simple sugars. Charred foods, excess salt, and certain food preservatives have been linked to diminished bone health, and should be avoided. Eating calcium-rich foods while avoiding foods that promote bone loss can help keep OP away. Heavy smoking and drinking are unhealthy habits at any age, and both have an effect on the body's nutritional intake. Cigarettes contain chemicals known to alter the way the body uses vitamin D, which normally boosts the body's ability to absorb calcium, meaning the calcium taken in by the organs might not be sufficient enough to prevent bone disease. Excessive drinking can also cause calcium loss and reduced levels of vitamin D. It's safe to say that a good prevention plan for OP involves avoiding cigarettes and alcohol as much as possible.[11]

Exercise is another very important factor in preventing OP. Remember that exercise and other physical activities increase bone strength, and when bones are stronger, OP can be avoided. Weight-bearing exercise, which helps strengthen bones, and aerobic exercise, which can help stabilize variable heart rate (VHR) in the long term, are both helpful in reducing the chances of developing OP. People approaching midlife should specifically focus on low-weight-bearing exercise. It is recommended that adults 19 to 60 years old get an hour of aerobic exercise per week to keep the bones healthy. For those aged 70 and above, 20 minutes per week is enough, and only if the doctor recommends it.[12]

The DXA test, discussed earlier, is advised for women 65 years and older and men aged 70 years and above. It measures a BMD, and when performed correctly, allows patients to know their current bone density and indicates whether they are at high risk of developing OP. Armed with this information, patients can already look for ways—as recommended by their doctor—to reverse or delay the condition. One factor in the prevention of OP is stress reduction. Under stress, the body releases a hormone called cortisol, which can impact bone health if present in the body at high levels. One effect of cortisol is lowering the ability of the digestive system to absorb calcium, causing the bones to lose strength and deteriorate. The impact of mental stress in patients and their caregivers shouldn't be underestimated, because it is usually much greater than expected. Knowing that stress can have this impact on bone health, it is clear that OP prevention must include ways to minimize stress. Simple ways to do this include laughing, meditating, drinking tea, spending time with friends, and just enjoying life.[13]

Recommendations for sleep may sound all too common, but getting adequate sleep really does have an impact when it comes to preventing OP. In its simplest form, sleep is when the body relaxes, grows, and repairs. Quality sleep helps strengthen the whole body, including the bones, and it is an essential factor in preventing OP. Caregivers and patients should know that sleep is when the body heals and recharges. For people undergoing treatment of musculoskeletal conditions, proper sleep is also a good way to return the body to its formerly healthy state, aside from the fact that well-rested organs and tissues can recover faster. This is true for practically any medical condition, not just OP. For those in the age range of 18 to 64 years, the recommended amount of sleep is between six to eight hours per day. Young adults and those age 65 years and older should check with their doctor to determine the ideal amount of sleep they should get each day. Osteoporosis patients might ask about sleep during their regular healthcare visits, another part of the preventive care plan that can help them avoid further illness.[14]

All these preventive tips can easily become regular activities that most people are already aware of. The important thing is to maintain consistent habits to keep the body healthy and reduce the risk of developing OP.

Prevention of OP Can Improve the Quality of Life of Other Bone Disorder Patients

Osteopenia is a condition clinically similar to OP but milder, as it involves the loss of minerals in the bones instead of the reduction of bone mass itself. People who are currently losing bone, as determined and validated by different tests, or who have risk factors for further bone thinning should be treated with lower doses of the same medications as people who have OP. Since it is so closely related to OP, osteopenia can be prevented using the same measures as those intended to prevent OP. Osteopenia can also be confirmed through a DEXA scan, which means that in addition to detecting OP, it can also determine the presence of osteopenia. Alas, a procedure intended to diagnose one condition can lead to the detection of another, and then the two medical conditions can be addressed as soon as possible.[15]

Osteomalacia is a bone condition much like OP, but it is caused by prolonged vitamin D deficiency. Vitamin D is essential for absorption of calcium throughout the body, from the person's guts all the way into the bloodstream. When calcium absorption is inadequate due to vitamin D deficiency, the cells and tissues won't have enough calcium to rebuild the skeleton. This leads to poorly calcified bone and shows the same clinical signs as OP. Diffuse bone pain as well as muscle aches may develop, and in severe cases osteomalacia leads to bone fractures, much like what can happen in OP. However, most osteomalacia patients have a mild form and are almost asymptomatic. Diagnosis is usually made during the investigation of low BMD results obtained by DXA scans. Like OP, osteomalacia can be prevented by increasing consumption of foods rich in vitamin D.[16]

Osteogenesis imperfecta, also called brittle bone disease, is a rare hereditary bone disease of connective tissue, characterized by brittle bones. Although it might not be completely prevented, preventive care for osteogenesis imperfecta also involves increased intake of calcium and vitamin D.[17]

Paget's disease of bone is different from OP in that a part of the skeleton, sometimes just one bone, suffers greatly from uncontrolled and irregular bone remodeling reshaping. When this happens, the affected bone is thickened, but nonetheless weakened. This irregular bone structure is easily observed on X-rays. Paget's patients may have pain in the affected bone or pain from the compression of neighboring nerves, and most often than not, the pain is very serious. Deformation of weight-bearing bones can be seen prominently in those affected with Paget's. Regrettably, medical scientists have yet to unearth the root cause of this condition, but the investigation is ongoing. Although this condition is highly different from OP, involving an increased but abnormal bone remodeling pathway, increased calcium intake can help keep the bones strong.[18]

ANALYSIS

By performing preventive actions, these OP and other musculo-skeletal conditions brought about by bone loss, lack of calcium, lack of vitamin D, and the like can be avoided. Increased intake of calcium-rich foods and vitamin D are important preventive measures. As with most medical conditions, preventive care plays a big role in mitigating the negative effects of OP, helping patients avoid medical procedures that will impact their lives in terms of time, energy, and money. Preventive care is crucial to helping people avoid developing critical and serious medical conditions that will keep them from living their lives to the fullest.[19]

Exercise and Osteoporosis

Physical activity has become a crucial aspect of a healthy lifestyle. People have different reasons for exercising, including minimizing the risk of stroke, keeping their blood sugar in check, and maintaining healthy weight. However, exercise can be even more helpful for OP patients, as it helps strengthen bones. As people age, their bones become weak and fragile, with or without OP. The presence of OP, however, increases the risk of broken bones that will ultimately limit their mobility. Exercise is therefore crucial to exercise to building and maintaining strong bones. Good habits around exercise should be built when people are young so that as they grow older, they can have already developed practices that will help maintain their bone strength. Exercise benefits the bones the same way it does the muscles: it makes them stronger. The more people exercise, the more dense their bones become as a result of the extra physical force. Eating right is not the only solution to the prevention and management of OP; exercise is necessary as well, especially exercises that strengthen bones and muscles. This chapter explores physical exercises that are good as well as bad for OP patients.[1]

SIGNIFICANCE OF EXERCISE

It is very important for premenopausal women to keep the BMD they achieved in their younger years in check. Estrogen aids in bone wellness by protecting against osteoclasts, or bone cells that disintegrate bones through resorption, and balancing bone turnover. When women with OP practice weight-bearing exercises regularly, estrogen and related female hormones help in maintaining strong bones and controls bone density. The joints also need motion in order to remain healthy. When they are left inactive for prolonged periods, it can lead to stiffening of the joint and weakening of the adjoining tissue. It is therefore important to do moderate exercises, although this is unlikely to slow the progression of OP. Those who stick to an exercise regimen, however, can reduce pain and disability.[2]

Osteoporosis patients with proper hormone health are better able to perform the tasks of daily life and are more likely than their inactive peers to remain independent in old age. However, it is always recommended that older individuals and anyone with a diagnosed medical condition to consult their physician before starting any exercise regimen. If the right exercise regimen is followed, it can help slow the advancement of OP and curtail the risk of falling, which normally results in fractures. Falls have been found to be among the leading causes of death in people over 65 years old. Exercise assists in building flexibility and equilibrium, ultimately lowering the risk of falling.[3]

Those OP patients who do not regularly exercise face the risk of suffering from low back pain. This mostly happens when they undertake stressful activities that require bending such as moving heavy things, tilling, or shoveling. While there is sufficient evidence to support the correlation between low back pain and lack of exercise, caregivers should note that sedentary living is most likely responsible for it. When someone with OP fails to exercise, they expose themselves to certain conditions that might have a negative impact on their backs. These include:

- *Obesity.* This condition exerts more weight on their spine, which in turn puts more pressure on their disks and vertebrae.
- *Muscle inflexibility.* This normally hinders the back's capability to bend, move, or rotate.
- *Weak back muscles.* This increases the duration of spinal pressure, which could lead to vertebral disk compression.
- *Weak stomach muscles.* This increases strain on the back, causing abnormal pelvis tilt.[4]

The key to enhancing flexibility lies in repetition, which helps build endurance as well as strengthening the bones.

THE REASONING BEHIND EXERCISE

Exercise can mitigate factors that contribute to poor bone health, including:

- *Gender.* Women are at a disadvantage when it comes to bone density; theirs is less than that of men, putting them at a higher risk of OP.
- *Inadequate calcium in the diet.* When people consume a diet low in calcium, they risk early bone loss and fractures due to low bone density.
- *Alcohol and tobacco use.* Tobacco use has been found to lead to weak bones. The same is true for excessive alcohol intake, which increases the risk of developing OP because alcohol inhibits calcium intake in the body.
- *Hormone levels.* An excess of thyroid hormone in the body can lead to bone loss. In women, this often happens after

they hit menopause as their estrogen levels dip. Those women who go for long periods without menstruating, such as during pregnancy, are also at a greater risk of OP, as are men with low testosterone levels.

- *Age.* As people grow older, their bones become weak and thin, thus increasing their risk of OP.

- *Physical activity.* Physically active people are at a lower risk for OP when compared to their inactive counterparts.

- *Size.* People with a BMI lower than 20 and those with small body frames are at a higher risk of OP, as they are likely to have less bone mass to draw from as they age.[5]

Several different types of exercises help with bone problems, while some do more harm than good. Before settling for a particular type of exercise, people with bone problems such as OP should consider what is best for their condition and what is clearly not. Some exercises are great, while others should be avoided, as the wrong kind of exercise can leave them in more pain than they had originally. Weight-bearing exercises signal the body to produce more tissue that helps in building stronger bones. Other exercises, including swimming, are good for the lungs and heart but do not help to ameliorate OP. Swimming and other water-related activities are not weight-bearing exercises since the buoyancy of the water counters the effect of gravity. However, water exercises can help in improving cardiovascular fitness and muscle strength. Patients with severe OP who are at high risk for fractures may find swimming and other water-related exercises to be their best option. The exercises most often recommended for people with OP are low-impact exercises. Osteoporosis patients are advised to consult their doctor before beginning any exercise regimen to ensure it is appropriate to their overall treatment plan.[6]

Best Exercises for Osteoporosis Pain/Chronic Bone Disease

There are many exercises that, when done the right way, can help OP patients rebuild their bones and minimize the risk of fractures.[7]

Osteoporosis patients need to not only build up their bones but also work their muscles. By doing this, they minimize the rate of bone density loss. Exercise can also help them forestall any fractures resulting from falls by way of muscle conditioning. These exercises can be as basic as standing on the toes to lifting the body weight through push-ups or squats. For exercises to be effective, OP patients should incorporate them into a workout regimen twice or three times a week. Some of the equipment that can help with such exercises includes:

- Free weights
- Exercise elastic bands
- Weight machines

Cardiovascular Conditioning and Weight-Bearing Exercises

Osteoporosis patients should take part in cardiovascular exercises that incorporate weight. This means that they should choose jogging, walking, or dancing instead of biking or swimming. They should also increase the exercise intensity, which can be achieved in several ways.[9]

Those looking to enhance their bone density should increase the intensity of their usual walking pace for short periods of time. Walking is a very effective weight-bearing exercise that helps in maintaining good general health, cardiac health, and muscle and bone health. The benefits derived from walking as exercise help reduce the risk of falling, which is a common cause of fractures. Studies have shown that walking helps to slow down the age-related reduction in bone density. Osteoporosis patients can also choose to climb up or down a hill, which will exert just the right amount of force on their bones. To make cardiovascular conditioning more effective, they should alternate higher-intensity and lower-intensity workouts. The trick is to go for at least two days of high-intensity workouts per week and alternate these with no fewer than four days of lower-intensity workouts.[10]

For those just starting out, it is best to gradually increase workout time until they are comfortable with 30 minutes of cardiovascular conditioning exercises each day for the best portion of the week. When it comes to weight-bearing workouts, experts suggest standing while doing them. This way, the bones and muscles work against the force of gravity, which is important in OP patients, and ensures they remain in an upright position. Bones tend to react to all the weight being placed on them by increasing bone building and in turn becoming sturdier. Osteoporosis patients should be wary of high-impact weight-bearing exercises, as some might not be safe for those who have a higher likelihood of fracturing a bone. Normally, OP patients are advised to opt for lower-impact exercises that do not pose the threat of bone fracture but still help in building up their bone density. Some of these include:

- Stair-step machines
- Walking
- Low-impact aerobics
- Cross-training machines

CLIMBING STAIRS AND LEG PRESSES

Exercise for OP patients can be as simple as moving up and down the stairs a few times, perhaps once in the morning and again in the evening. Climbing stairs provides the entire lower body with an effective workout. It helps create lean, strong leg muscles because it uses all the muscles in the leg, including hamstrings, glutes, calves, and quadriceps. This exercise puts a bit more stress on muscles and joints, making them stronger. It is a good exercise for people with OP, especially those who cannot run due to pain and stiffness. Leg presses are done by pushing some weight or resistance away from the body using the legs. This exercise has an immense effect on one's skeleton. It exerts pressure and stress on the bones, which in turn makes them strong. When done in moderation, this is an ideal exercise for OP patients, as the amount of force applied is up to the individual. Elliptical training (simulating stair climbs) is a low-impact weight-bearing exercise good for people with OP. This type of exercise offers low stress on the joints and helps improve balance, coordination, and muscle strength.[12]

STRETCHING EXERCISES

Stretching exercises are also ideal for people with OP. By lengthening all their tight muscles, they can minimize back pain and improve the mechanics of their spine as well as their posture. The muscles in the body that commonly stiffen are those used to arch the back, those responsible for lifting, knees, external rotators and shoulder elevators, and ankle dorsiflexors. Osteoporosis patients should slowly stretch to a point they are comfortable, without any pain or overexertion. Stretching exercises are most beneficial when performed once or twice a day.[13]

NONIMPACT EXERCISES

Although nonimpact exercises may not make the bones tougher, they do help OP patients enhance their coordination, muscle strength, and flexibility. This is very important, as it helps in lowering the likelihood of bone-related injuries. These exercises can also be done every day without exerting too much pressure on the bones. One helpful balance exercise is tai chi, which helps increase flexibility and improves balance. These posture workouts are also ideal for helping patients correct shoulder sloping that is common in OP and help lower the risk of spine fracture. Tai chi is a low-impact activity that is safe for OP patients, as it does not put the joints and bones at risk. Studies have shown that tai chi helps in improving muscle strength, coordination, and balance as well as reducing pain and stiffness in the muscles and joints.[14]

Other ideal nonimpact exercises include Pilates and yoga, which help improve balance, strength, and flexibility. However, some yoga and Pilates routines could prove harmful for OP patients, including forward-bending moves, as they expose patients to the risk of bone breakage. Osteoporosis patients should then talk to their doctor before beginning these exercises so they can be advised which moves are safe for them and which are not. Practicing yoga is especially beneficial to people with OP because studies have shown that yoga can actually increase bone density if done properly and consistently. It also improves balance and flexibility, which is key in preventing falls and fractures. As a low-impact exercise, it is appropriate for people with OP and can in fact help lessen the pain associated with this condition. Certain poses that direct some body weight onto the hands may aid in the retention of body density in the upper extremities and backbone.[15]

FOOT STOMPS

When it comes to exercising to deal with OP, the goal should be to challenge the body parts affected by the condition, including the hips. Patients can challenge their hip bones by practicing foot stomps. These are normally practiced while standing. Patients perform the exercise by stomping their feet while imagining they are trying to squash a small tin can. This should be repeated at least four times on one foot before repeating the process on the other. Those who find it hard to balance can hold on to a sturdy piece of furniture or a railing.[16]

HAMSTRING CURLS

Hamstring curls strengthen the back of the upper legs and should always be done while standing. They are performed by standing with the legs apart and firmly planted, then trying to move the left foot so that only the toes are in contact with the ground. The next step involves contracting the back of the leg muscles to lift the left heel toward the buttocks. Then the leg is slowly lowered to the original position and the process repeated with the right leg. This exercise should be repeated up to 12 times a day.[17]

WEIGHTLIFTING

Weightlifting can help in preventing and managing OP-related fractures. Studies have shown that when done over a long period of time, weightlifting with dumbbells can aid in preventing bone loss and may even build new bones while fortifying existing ones. Maintaining strong bones and muscles through weightlifting improves coordination and stability, which is a key factor in preventing falls. Osteoporosis patients are advised to focus on the back and hips. Examples of the best exercises for OP patients include, but are not limited to: hip extension, hip abduction and adduction, and hip flexion—in other words, anything that works around the hip.[18]

Bicep Curls

People with OP can do bicep curls using either dumbbells weighing between one and five pounds or resistance bands. These exercises can be done while standing or sitting, whatever position patients find comfortable. To effectively do this, patients should hold a dumbbell in each hand or grasp an end of a resistance band in each hand while stepping on the band itself. They should then pull these weights or the band toward their chest while keeping an eye on the flexing bicep muscles before letting down the hands to the initial position. This process should be repeated for at least eight times before resting for a while and then performing a second set.

As the name suggests, a resistance band adds resistance to exercise, creating tension that causes the muscles to contract. This added resistance helps in strengthening the muscles as well as the bones. Caregivers can help by holding one end of the resistance band in place. The more the band is stretched, the more intense the resistance and the better for the bones and muscles. Resistance bands help in working out the muscle and bones, just like weight training does.[19]

Shoulder Lifts

Shoulder lifts also require a resistance band or weights, and can be performed either sitting down or standing. Just like with bicep curls, patients should either use dumbbells or stand on the resistance band while holding its ends. Starting with the hands down resting at their sides, they slowly should raise their arms in front of them, keeping them straight and taking care not to lock their elbows. The next step is lifting shoulders to a comfortable height, no higher than shoulder level. This exercise should be done up to 12 times before resting and then performing a second set if they are able to.[20]

OTHER EXERCISES

Ball Sit

As the name suggests, the ball sit exercise requires the use of a medicine ball. It is ideal for strengthening the abdominal muscles as well as improving balance. Patients should have a spotter to help them effectively balance their body while doing this exercise. The exercise is performed by sitting on the medicine ball with the feet firmly on the ground. The back should remain very straight to maintain balance, and if possible, the hands should be stretched out with the palms facing forward. This position should be held for up to 60 seconds before standing up to rest and then repeated once or twice more.[21]

Hip Leg Lifts

Hip leg lifts are ideal for strengthening the muscles surrounding the hips while improving balance, which is important for OP patients. Patients should steady themselves by holding onto a piece of furniture. They should then place their feet apart on the floor, hip width apart, and shift their weight to their left foot. Flexing their right foot while keeping it straight, they should lift it at least six inches from solid ground before lowering it. This should be repeated up to 12 times before returning the leg to the starting position and switching to the other leg to repeat the process.[22]

Squats

Squats are ideal for strengthening both the gluteus muscles and the front of the legs. It is not necessary to squat too far down in order to benefit from this exercise. Patients should begin with their feet apart while resting their hands on a piece of furniture for balance. The next step is to gently bend the knees into a squatting position while ensuring that the back remains straight, leaning forward slightly while squatting until the thighs are parallel to the floor, then tightening the buttock muscles before returning to a standing position. The exercise should be repeated at least eight times. Overall, this exercise helps in strengthening the muscles around the hip and the bones in the same area. This helps in enhancing balance, as the bones and the muscles around the hip support the weight of the upper part of the body. A few squats per day can work miracles for OP patients. It is not a rigorous exercise and therefore doesn't strain the body.[23]

Pushups

Pushups are a very common calisthenic exercise that begins by resting on the ground with the weight on the feet and hands and arms straightened. By using the arms to raise and lower the body, pushups work out the pectoral muscles, triceps, and anterior deltoids. They help in building upper-body strength, and done correctly, they help strengthen the lower back and core by pulling in the abdominal muscles. Pushups are a fast and effective type of exercise that help improve posture in people with OP.[24]

WORST EXERCISES FOR OP/CHRONIC PAIN/CHRONIC BONE DISEASE

Exercise is helpful in increasing and maintaining bone health in people with low bone density, but some exercises can be harmful. Some of the exercises they should avoid include:

• Those that require bending forward from the waist, as they are likely to lead to spine fractures

• Those that require hunching or rounding of the back

• Any pose that exerts weight on the neck

• Any spine-twisting movement that causes strain while either seated or standing

• Lifting heavy things

• Any rapid jerking movements

• Any activity that requires jumping, intense golfing or tennis, or dancing

Although many people find golf and tennis to be enjoyable outdoor games, they're not ideal for people with OP. This is because of the sudden twisting of the spine, resulting in extra force on discs and joints that could lead to fractures.[25]

Abdominal Exercises

Sit-ups are considered one of the best exercises to achieve a flat abdomen and a strong core, and many people perform them regularly. However, people with OP are normally advised to avoid doing sit-ups because they put too much pressure on the lower back, which could lead to lumbar spine fractures. Because people with OP often already have tiny fractures in their joints, the forward rounding of the spine can exacerbate the damage, resulting in an awkward "question mark" posture that is often present in people suffering from severe OP. They should opt instead for other exercises that don't stress the lumbar spine.[26]

Russian twists, which are a part of Pilates or high-intensity training, are not ideal for OP patients since they involve a lot of spine twisting and bending. These exercises involve the spine's full flexion as well as rotation. The lumbar spine vertebra can rotate up to three degrees, but these exercises take this to its end range, which is bad for the back. Another problem is caused by the standing side bend, which puts excessive force on the spine and could lead to fractures.[27]

Lumbar rolls are a popular yoga pose performed by laying on the back with knees held close to the chest, then rolling forward and backward slowly along the spine. The problem with this pose is that it introduces forward flexion to the spine, which could lead to further pain in the long run. Osteoporosis patients should therefore avoid it at all costs.[28]

Jumping Exercises

People with OP need to keep their feet on the ground most of the time. However, this is not the case when performing jumping exercises such as tuck jumps, jump squats, power planks, and pike jumps. These exercises break down bone and irritate the spine. Jumping normally bends the spine while putting pressure on the adjoining joints, so OP patients should avoid jumping exercises.

An alternative to intense jumping exercises that is safe for OP patients is jumping rope, which helps increase bone density. This exercise helps prevent OP by promoting bone growth and safely strengthening the joints. When someone jump ropes, they don't have to jump that high to avoid swiping the bottom of their feet with the rope. This is a simple exercise that can be done every day and doesn't strain the whole body.[29]

Skiing

Skiing is one of the many activities that expose participants to the risk of falling and should therefore be avoided by people with OP. The motion from these activities also leads to a lot of twisting. Since OP patients have an increased risk of fractures, any activity that has a high risk of falling should be avoided at all costs.

Skiing can be helpful in preventing OP, however, because it strengthens bones and joints. When moving downhill, the knees endure tension and weight from the body which makes them stronger. The weight-bearing impact on the legs helps make the bones and joints a lot more agile.[30]

ANALYSIS

Exercise is essential for people with OP, as it improves bone health. When starting off, patients should incorporate both muscle-strengthening and weight-bearing workouts, taking care to ensure that their bones can handle the exercises they choose. People with OP should always consult their doctor for advice about which exercises are safe and appropriate to their treatment plan. Doing the right exercises while avoiding unsafe ones is fundamental to managing OP. While physical exercises are useful managing OP, they can be harmful if not performed correctly. High-impact exercises are not safe for those with fragile bones.[31]

Bypassing Trigger Diets

THE HUMAN BODY REQUIRES A PARTICULAR LEVEL OF ENERGY and nutrients to function normally. Deficiency of certain nutrients in the diet leads to specific physiological disorders; for example, a diet that lacks vitamin D causes rickets, a lack of iron causes anemia, while scurvy is caused by a lack of vitamin C. Especially for OP patients, a proper diet is crucial for healthy living and requires foods that provide the right amount of energy and nutrients for optimal functioning. Experts advise those with conditions like OP to eat a proper diet because it helps them recover quickly. The right diet provides the body with energy, helps the body fight chronic (long-term) illnesses, and relieves the symptoms and discomfort observed in chronic illnesses.[1]

THE IMPORTANCE OF PROPER DIET IN ALL MEDICAL CONDITIONS

Some of the foods known to have general health properties include the following:

- *Coconut water.* People with OP need to stay hydrated. Coconut water contains electrolytes and glucose, which help the body rehydrate.

- *Garlic.* Garlic stimulates immunity and fights viruses and bacteria, aiding in recovery from illness.

- *Broth.* Soup made of a mixture of meat and vegetables helps the body remain hydrated. Broth contains important minerals such as calcium, phosphorus, and magnesium. It also has some vitamins and calories, as well as high levels of nutrients and proteins. When consumed warm, the steam of broth acts as a natural decongestant.

- *Chicken soup.* Like broth, chicken soup helps keep patients hydrated and acts as a decongestant. It contains proteins, vitamins, and minerals.

- *Honey.* This amazing natural substance contains an antimicrobial compound that gives it a powerful antibacterial effect. It boosts the immune system and suppresses coughs.

- *Ginger.* Ginger has anti-inflammatory and antioxidant effects. It also helps to reduce nausea, boosts the immune system, and helps slow down the hardening of arteries, which in turn lowers blood pressure.

- *Citrus fruits.* These delicious fruits—including lemons, oranges, and grapefuit—are rich in vitamin C, which is known to increase production of the white blood cells that fight diseases.

- *Red bell peppers.* Red bell peppers have even higher levels of vitamin C than citrus fruits. Peppers contain beta-carotene, which boosts the immune system and maintains eye and skin health.

- *Broccoli.* Broccoli is among the healthiest items on any menu. It's an excellent source of vitamins A, C, and E and also contains fiber and many antioxidants.

- *Bananas.* These yellow delicacies are calorie-dense and rich in nutrients. They are easy to eat and swallow once their thick skin is peeled off, and their soluble fiber helps prevent diarrhea and reduce nausea.

- *Spinach.* This leafy green is rich in vitamin C. It also contains beta-carotene and numerous antioxidants that can fortify the immune system. When cooking, one cooks it lightly to boost its vitamin A content and other nutrient levels.

- *Yogurt.* Some yogurts contain probiotics beneficial to both children and adults. Yogurt promotes gut health and contains vitamin D, which helps regulate the immune system and boost the body's natural defense against illness.[2]

Facing Challenges to Healthy Eating

When people are ill, they tend to lose their appetite. Some are unable to cook on their own, while others have a problem swallowing the food. Some experience vomiting and nausea after eating. Regardless of the situation, a proper diet is vital to recovery. Proper diet boosts immunity and provides energy for peak body functioning.

The following strategies may help OP patients regain lost appetite:

- Consider eating smaller, more frequent meals.
- Reduce fluid intake before a meal. A lot of fluids make one feel full, which impacts appetite.
- Make mealtime enjoyable by eating favorite healthy meals accompanied by some cool music.
- Make it a habit to eat at a certain time.[3]

People with OP who have difficulty cooking on their own have several options:

- Stock up on fruits, vegetables, and fresh juice. Fruits and vegetables provide the body with many crucial nutrients.
- Get help from people who can supply ready food.
- Consult a nutritionist for advice.[4]

Osteoporosis patients who experience nausea and vomiting right after eating can keep the following in mind:

- Research indicates that crystallized ginger can help reduce nausea and vomiting, but ginger ale should be avoided as it can worsen an upset stomach.
- Pasta, rice, certain teas, and foods rich in protein are good options for fighting nausea.

Patients who have difficulty swallowing food (dysphagia) can also take fluids such as soup, energy drinks, fruit juice, and milk to stay hydrated throughout the day. However, they should avoid fluids that cause dehydration, such as alcohol and caffeine. Patients with active wounds should eat foods high in protein, which helps to heal tissues. Carbohydrates, fat, vitamins, and minerals are also essential to speed up the healing process.[5]

THE BEST DIETS FOR OP/CHRONIC PAIN/CHRONIC BONE DISEASE

The body requires a combination of calcium, magnesium, manganese, and phosphorus to build strong bones. Lack of one or all of these critical nutrients may cause chronic bone disease, so a proper diet for OP patients must contain these nutrients. Diet is a crucial factor in fighting OP. A balanced diet contains the right amounts of proteins, fats, carbohydrates, vitamins, minerals, fiber, and water. These amounts vary depending on the age and general wellness of the individual. Doctors suggest that at breakfast, OP patients should consume food and drinks rich in calcium and vitamin D to begin the day strong. Throughout the day, portions of calcium and vitamin D should be spread throughout all their meals to improve calcium absorption. Doctors recommend that every day, adults with OP should take in around 1500mg of calcium. Foods that are good sources of calcium include soybeans, tofu, nuts, bread made with calcium-fortified wheat, broccoli, cabbage, okra, and some fish such as sardines. Vitamin D is activated by the sun and is found in food and supplements. People younger than age 70 should take 600 International Units (IU) daily, while those older than 70 should take 800 IU per day. Natural sources of vitamin D include eggs, some powdered milk varieties, low-fat butter spread, breakfast cereals, and oily fish such as sardines and mackerel. Supplements containing vitamin D are recommended for OP patients who do not get enough in their diet.[6]

People at risk of vitamin D deficiency include:

- Babies and children under age four
- Individuals with dark skin
- People who wear clothing that covers the whole body while outdoors
- People who are naturally frail since birth
- Confined/incarcerated individuals
- Vegetarians[7]

People who don't eat any meat can get the vitamins their bodies need from dried fruits such as raisins, tofu, and fortified soy. They can get vitamin D by exposing their skin to sunshine and taking vitamin D supplements.

SUPERFOODS FOR OP PATIENTS

People with OP should eat plenty of fruits and vegetables, especially ones like spinach, bananas, oranges, papaya, and collard greens. These contain important substances such as phytochemicals that improve the health of people suffering from OP. They are also high in fiber and contain vitamins A, C, and K, as well as essential minerals such as potassium and magnesium that help to maintain healthy bones. Prunes are especially good for postmenopausal women with OP, since they can help prevent and reverse bone loss. They contain vitamin C, which slows the progression of disease by boosting the immune system and preventing cartilage loss.[8]

Organic full-fat yogurt, available in a variety of flavors, contains many beneficial nutrients important to the bones, including calcium, magnesium, zinc, vitamin A, vitamin D, and a small amount of vitamin K2. Yogurt also helps the bones absorb nutrients and improves digestion because it is full of healthy probiotic bacteria that establish themselves in the intestines and help protect the gut. Probiotic bacteria provide vitamin B to support healthy bones and energy metabolism. These microorganisms also support the nervous system and the cardiovascular system. A cup of organic yogurt daily provides the body with proteins, calcium, and vitamin D3. In contrast to organic yogurt, inorganic yogurt lacks fat-soluble vitamins A and K2. It may also contain hormones, antibiotic residue, and pesticide residue, along with a variety of chemical additives and GMO sugars. All of these can be harmful to the bones.[9]

People with OP can get proteins from foods such as meat, chicken, lentils, eggs, and milk. Protein helps the body recover from daily wear and tear and is essential for strong muscles. For those who do not eat meat, lentils, soybeans, and rice can be combined to make a meal rich in protein. Beans, peas and chicken help in the building of bone density. Cooked lentils also help to control blood sugar and blood pressure. Bone broth is rich in proline and glycine amino acids, which make up certain proteins. It is also full of minerals such as calcium, magnesium, and phosphorus, and contains vitamins and antioxidants that help in maintaining healthy bones.[10]

Fermented foods contain vitamin K, which helps in preserving bone density and is known to help form blood clots in crucial times in hemophiliacs. Vitamin K creates a balance between osteoblasts (the cells that break down bones) and osteoclasts (the cells that build bones). Fermented foods include yogurt, kefir, kombucha, and natto.[11]

Turmeric, a common spice used in cooking, has anti-inflammatory properties vital in treating OP and rheumatoid arthritis. It has a distinctive color as a result of a high concentration of curcumin, which helps to reduce muscle damage.[12]

Green tea supports bone health by offering nutritional support. It contains anti-inflammatory compounds known as flavonoids as well as catechins or polyphenols, which are powerful antioxidants. Since one of the major contributing factors to bone loss is oxidative stress, consuming green tea is important. Anti-inflammatory compounds and antioxidants help the bones to stay strong and healthier. Regular intake of green and black tea increases mineral density.[13]

UNFAVORABLE DIETS FOR PEOPLE WITH OP

Some common foods contribute to OP and should be avoided. The standard American diet (SAD) is associated with OP risk because it is high in refined sugars and carbohydrates that gradually destroy bones and is heavy in foods that lack essential minerals such as calcium and vitamins that are building blocks of healthy bones. SAD lacks high-nutrient food such as vegetables and legumes. Many of the foods it contains cause chronic inflammation and metabolic acidosis, a condition in which the body's pH becomes acidic, leaching calcium from the bones. Many of the food and drinks common in SAD should be avoided by OP patients.[14]

Carbonated beverages such as sodas are associated with lower bone mineral density. These drinks contain phosphorus, an essential mineral for OP patients; however, when consumed in large amounts, it produces phosphoric acid, which is harmful to the bones. Excessive phosphorus levels leach calcium from the bones, and the body expels it through the urine. Full-sugar and sugar-free sodas both have the same effect. Moreover, excessive consumption of the caffeine found in most carbonated soft drinks is harmful to postmenopausal women. It reduces their bone density and energy by leaching calcium from the bones. Experts note that for every 100mg of caffeine consumed, about 6mg of calcium is lost. Beans contain calcium, magnesium, and fiber—known to be useful in the body—that helps in the prevention of OP.[15]

There's a strong link between OP and excessive vitamin A (retinol). Foods containing vitamin A, such as salmon, may be consumed in small quantities, but people with OP should limit their intake of retinol to less than 1.5 mg per day and should also avoid supplements containing too much retinol. Raw spinach and Swiss chard are helpful to the body since they provide the right amount of retinol. Unfortunately, they also have oxalates that bind calcium compounds together, making the calcium unavailable to be used by the body. These greens should be consumed in combination with other foods such as cheese, which contains readily absorbable calcium.[16]

Inflammatory foods are foods that can cause inflammation—a response to injury or irritation—in the body. Inflammatory foods are not healthy for OP patients and can cause OP. In fact, one of the main causes of OP is prolonged inflammation in the body. Inflammatory foods are found in many different types of international cuisine, but some of the most common inflammatory foods are red meat, dairy products, and processed foods. Inflammatory foods have been linked to a number of health problems, including OP. The inflammation caused by such foods can lead to bone loss and an increased risk for fractures.[17]

People with OP should keep their sodium levels in check. They should avoid overconsumption of prepacked or fast-food French fries, as they are usually sprinkled with large amounts of salt. Postmenopausal women who consume a lot of salt lose BMD at a higher rate than their age would otherwise suggest. Excess salt weakens bones over time. Researchers have found that excess salt exacerbates hypertension and causes more calcium to be expelled through the urine. Assuming all this calcium is from the bones, that translates to 1 percent bone loss annually. People with OP should consume a diet low in salt, preferably less than 5g per day. Some foods and fluids that should be avoided include salad dressing, canned foods, bagels, frozen dinners, and soft drinks. These should be replaced with organic yogurt, dark leafy greens, dried fruits, tea, coconut, unsalted rice water, pasta, and fresh fish. Those who are unable to reduce their salt intake should supplement their diet with foods rich in potassium, such as bananas, tomatoes, and orange juice, which can help to decrease the loss of calcium.[18]

Excessive alcohol consumption is harmful to the body. Scientists have determined that consuming red wine moderately on a regular basis has positive benefits for bone health. Red wine contains resveratrol, which is helpful to bone-resorbing osteoclasts and formation of bone-building osteoblasts. Female OP patients should drink half a glass of wine or beer daily, and men, a full glass. However, excessive consumption of alcohol increases the chances of bone fracture and slows the healing of broken bones. It also causes low bone mass and decreased bone formation. Female patients who begin consuming alcohol at a younger age have lower bone density than those who begin at an older age. Alcoholics should minimize their consumption of alcohol to just one or two glasses a day.[19]

Osteoporosis patients with food sensitivities are likely to have chronic inflammation that damages the bones through indirect physiological pathways. Chronic inflammation within the digestive system is caused by a leaky gut, in which the intestinal lining allows toxins and undigested food to pass from the intestines into the open areas of the abdominal cavity. This triggers an immune response in the form of chronic inflammation. This problem affects a huge number of people globally. Symptoms of food sensitivities include bowel issues, indigestion, and possibly flatulence and reflux. It is advisable that people who notice these signs try to discover the cause by eliminating the food suspected of causing it and monitoring symptoms over a period of a few days or weeks. They should also visit the doctor for a sensitivity test.[20]

There are different categories of fats. Some fats are useful to the body, while others are very harmful. One kind of healthy fat is omega-3 fatty acids, which are found in fish, dairy, and avocados as well as in oils such as olive and flaxseed. Healthy fats boost energy and helps in the transportation of soluble vitamins like A, D, E, and K, which help the body to absorb calcium. Vegetable oils such as corn, sunflower, and canola contain polyunsaturated omega-6 fatty acids, which is an unhealthy fat. Unlike omega-3, which is anti-inflammatory, omega-6 encourages inflammation. Most harmful fats are trans fats, which promote inflammation, reduce HDL cholesterol, and increase LDL cholesterol, increasing the risk of heart problems and chronic inflammation. They are also associated with causing insulin sensitivity, cancer, obesity, and OP. Trans fats are found in processed food, fries, chips, and cookies. Although it is important to avoid trans fats, people with OP should keep in mind the importance of healthy fats in boosting energy and absorbing fat-soluble vitamins, aiming to get about 20 to 35 percent of their calories from sources of healthy fats.[21]

Carbohydrates and refined sugars are two things that cannot be ignored when it comes to OP triggers. Consumption of excess sugar has been associated with diseases such as gout and high blood pressure as well as damage to vital organs such as the liver and heart. Carbohydrates and refined sugars also deplete minerals and vitamins and raise LDL cholesterol. Excess consumption of sugar can also raise triglyceride levels, which, along with high LDL cholesterol, can cause fat to build up around artery walls, increasing the risk of stroke or heart attack in people with and without OP. Excess sugar consumption can contribute to weight gain and insulin resistance that causes type 2 diabetes. It also triggers inflammation that causes aging of skin and damage to the bones. This inflammation is caused by glycation and later accelerated by high blood sugar. Glycation is an attachment of glucose to collagen and elastin proteins that makes the resulting compound very rigid. At advanced levels, glycation results in advanced glycation end products (AGEs) and it is a cause of conditions such as Alzheimer's and Parkinson's disease. High blood sugar levels are harmful to the bones because they result in massive loss of calcium through the urine. Digested carbohydrates easily convert into glucose, so foods like cakes and cookies should be avoided. Because of the complications that can be caused by excessive intake of refined sugars, OP patients should use natural sugars such as raw honey and stevia. People with OP should also avoid foods such as soda, bread, chips, bagels, biscuits, cakes, and canned soup, all of which contain high levels of glucose—some up to 100mg per serving. These should be replaced with foods like lentils, seafood, pumpkin seeds, and almonds.[22]

Advanced glycation end products are also present in over-cooked or charred food. Antioxidants and enzymes help the body to eliminate AGEs, but the body can't keep up if AGEs increase rapidly. Once the body is unable to handle the surge, a strong inflammation response is triggered. Proper cooking technique is vital in order to eliminate extra AGEs in the food. Instead of high-heat cooking, foods should be cooked at medium-high temperatures. People with OP should avoid baking, broiling, and toasting foods, and instead opting for boiling, steaming, or slow cooking. Highly processed foods and items rich in animal fats and proteins—such as red meat, fried eggs, and cheese—should not be consumed in excess as they contain high levels of AGEs.[23]

ANALYSIS

Proper diet plays a major role in either causing, preventing, or healing OP. Everyone needs food containing calcium, vitamin D, and other healthy substances to ensure good health. Proper diet helps to stop bone fracture and speed the healing process. People with OP should consult their doctor to determine an appropriate diet and get food supplements if need be.[24]

13

Alternative versus Conventional Approaches

THE MAJOR GOAL OF ANY KIND OF ALTERNATIVE TREATMENT IS to manage or heal the condition. Although there is not absolute, concrete, scientific, or clinical proof to suggest that they are *always* effective, the majority of people who use these methods report success. Before trying any kind of medication, it is always advisable to try natural methods, since there are no side effects and natural remedies do not contain man-made chemicals that might later be determined to have a negative impact on health. There are a variety of alternative methods that are useful in managing OP.[1]

USE OF SUPPLEMENTS

The foods people eat contain an assortment of nutrients, minerals, and other critical ingredients that assist in keeping the body sound. Specific supplements are often required for bone strength and the health of the heart, muscles, and nerves. The use of supplements is a natural way to improving the immune system and a cost-effective way to handle many health conditions, as some medications deplete essential nutrients in the body as well as the finances. The most recommended supplements for OP are ones containing the following:

- *Calcium.* This is the most important mineral patients can take to manage OP. It helps in maintaining the bone mass required to support the skeleton. It is also necessary for healthy muscle, nerve, and heart function. Strong bones reduces the chances of the fractures associated with OP.

- *Vitamin D.* Calcium should be taken together with vitamin D for effective results. This is because vitamin D helps in the absorption of calcium in building strong bones. Vitamin D is not naturally found in any foods or supplements, but it is cultivated through sun exposure. However, vitamin D2 and vitamin D3 are available in the form of supplements and they are equally helpful in building and strengthening bones.

- *Magnesium.* This supplement assures bone durability. Magnesium and calcium work hand in hand, a deficiency of one affects the metabolism of the other. Simply put, an increase in calcium without a proportionate increase in magnesium can lead to a loss of magnesium. Similarly, the use of calcium in the presence of magnesium deficiency can result in calcium deposits in the soft tissues such as joints, causing bone and joint problems.

- *Vitamin K.* This supplement is necessary because it helps in fusing calcium into the bones. It also helps keep calcium in the bones. Therefore, calcium cannot be effective in the total absence of vitamin K.

- *Boron.* Boron is a necessary mineral that helps the body to effectively utilize calcium. It also has properties that help in OP treatment through activation of minerals and vitamins necessary for bone formation and development.

- *Silicon.* Silicon helps in the development of healthy bones, ligaments, and tendons. Like boron, it is a trace mineral, but it plays a crucial role in building and stabilizing bones.

- *Strontium.* This is a powerful mineral utilized in treatment and prevention of OP. The mineral is found in water and food, and it can be traced in the human skeleton, where it is present in the crystal surfaces of the bone.

- *Melatonin.* This is a hormone produced by the pineal gland in the brain. It is usually associated with sleep and plays a very important role in maintaining and improving bone density, especially in old age. Melatonin is believed to increase the activity of bone-building osteoblasts and influences the thickening of bones when necessary.[2]

Herbal Products

The use of herbal products is the most economical and convenient method of preventing and managing OP. This is because these products are readily available and are not expensive. They contain no added chemicals thus avoid the associated health risks. There are several common herbs used to manage OP:

- *Red Clover.* It has been scientifically proven that red clover can prevent OP. Studies have shown that the most common type of OP is usually linked to ovarian hormonal deficiency, particularly during menopause. Red clover contains estrogen-like compounds. Therefore, a diet with high levels of phyto-estrogenic isoflavones (an example of estrogen-like compounds) reduces risk of OP and other menopause-related complications. Red clover also aids in bone healing and internal bone mineralization steps that maintain bone density.

- *Soy.* Products such as soybeans, soy milk, and tofu are good sources of proteins and calcium. Soy products are bone-friendly additions to any meal. In fact, soybeans contain all the eight most essential minerals. Soy is also a rich source of isoflavones, which, just like human estrogen, have a beneficial effect on bones.

- *Black Cohosh.* Black cohosh contains estrogen-like substances called phytoestrogens, which prevents bone loss. The herb also promotes bone formation and thus reduces the risk of OP.

- *Horsetail.* Horsetail contains silicon, a very strong mineral that helps to counter bone loss by stimulating bone regeneration. Its consumption helps in increasing bone density.

- *Fruits and vegetables.* Most fruits and vegetables contain the most essential vitamins and minerals such as magnesium, calcium, potassium, vitamin K, vitamin C, as well as proteins that are essential for strong bones. Edible plants contain anti-inflammatory and antioxidant agents, which are very effective in countering inflammation and oxidative stress. It's been scientifically proven that high intake of fruits and vegetables aids in increasing bone mass.[3]

ALTERNATIVE APPROACHES

Acupuncture is a form of treatment in which a thin needle is inserted through the skin at a specific point on the body and at given depths. This helps in balancing hormones and other internal energetic imbalances that contribute to the loss of bone mass. Acupuncture is very effective in alleviating OP-related pain and aids in improving bone density. Acupuncture is beneficial because it is safe, has very few side effects, can effectively be used alongside other treatments, controls pain, and is ideal for the patients who react poorly to pain medications. It is not, however, recommended for patients with bleeding disorders.[4]

Massage can be very useful for OP patients, but it is important to note that not all massages are recommended. For patients with severe OP, it has to be a light massage that's not going to strain the body. Massage has many specific benefits for OP patients:

- *Relaxation.* A light massage is the perfect way to relaxing the muscles and joints, improving flexibility.

- *Freedom of movement.* A well-administered massage improves joint movement, which in turn brings steadiness of the bones. Range of motion is also improved as the joints become more flexible.

- *Posture.* For the patients whose posture has been adversely affected by OP or a related condition, a slight massage is administered regularly over a long period can correct or reverse the condition.

- *Pain relief.* Massage is a great way to relieve pain associated with OP and other medical conditions. Pain relief is achieved through muscle and tissue relaxation that reduces painful contractions and nerve compression.

- *Increased joint health.* Massage therapists also massage joints to make them strong enough to support the bones. Healthy joints mean healthy bones, and this is all that an OP patient requires.[5]

The following massages are recommended for patients with musculoskeletal disorders:

- *Swedish massage.* This type of massage achieves relaxation through a combination of movements such as muscle kneading and rolling; long, sweeping strokes; and friction. The massage starts and ends with long, sweeping strokes, with muscle kneading being administered throughout to help in working out tensed muscle, while friction may be applied with fingertips on muscles requiring deeper pressure. This kind of massage is great for full body relaxation and for patients with injuries or bone-related conditions.

- *Hot stone massage.* This type of massage is administered by placing smooth, hot stones on specific points on the back. The massage therapist then uses the stones to massage the patient. The heated stones release tension in the shoulders and the back, while the massage helps relax the entire body. This type of massage is mostly used for relaxation.

- *Aromatherapy massage.* Aromatherapy massage can be a great option for pain relief. The aroma itself triggers the mind into relaxation, helping fight pain.[6]

When administering massage to OP patients, the following should be taken into consideration:

- The client should be positioned comfortably.
- A pillow should be placed under the trunk or back and the cervical spine.
- Excess pressure should be avoided.
- Flexion and high-impact exercises should be avoided.[7]

CONVENTIONAL TREATMENT METHODS FOR OP

In severe cases of OP, healthy behaviors may not completely offset bone loss either due to age or illness. This is where prescription medication comes in. There has been a lot of research that has led to the development of drugs that have rendered OP treatable. However, in less severe cases, as noted above, it is always advisable to seek alternative methods first; if no improvement is noted after a few weeks, then one can seek pharmacological intervention. In recent years, advancements in the field of medicine have made it possible to get more insight into the biology of the bones. This has made possible the development of various pharmaceutical methods of treating and preventing OP. Parathyroid hormone, potent bisphosphonates, derivatives of vitamin D, calcitonin, selective estrogen receptor modulators, and estrogen replacement therapy are just a few of the approved OP pharmacological therapies. Bone loss can be prevented by the use of these drugs (except parathyroid hormones) because most of these drugs act as antiresorptive agents.[8]

These drugs are also associated with increasing the bone density while at the same time reducing the risk of bone fractures. Alendronate (Fosamax), an OP medication, significantly improves BMD, reducing the risk of fracture by between 12 and 28 percent. However, in patients suffering from OP, the use of alendronate reduces the risk of fracture occurrence substantially. While most patients experience some therapeutic benefit from the available treatments, the fact remains that there is no treatment that completely eliminates the risk of fractures. Some patients experience no effect or negative effects from treatment, and there is no way to determine in advance the effect—positive, negative, or none at all—a treatment will have on a particular patient.[9]

Several conventional approaches are available for the prevention and treatment of OP, including bisphosphonates, calcitonin, estrogen (hormone treatment), estrogen agonists/enemies (SERMs), parathyroid hormone, parathyroid hormone-related protein (PTHrp), RANK ligand (RANKL) inhibitor, and tissue-selective estrogen complex (TSEC).[10]

Denosumab (Prolia) is a monoclonal antibody used to treat bone loss in women with an increased risk of breaking bones following menopause. Other drugs used for treatment or management of OP are bisphosphonates, which include alendronate (Fosamax) and risedronate (Actonel), which are taken either daily or weekly. Ibandronate (Boniva) is used on a monthly basis for treatment and prevention of OP. Zoledronic acid (Reclast) is taken intravenously once a year for treatment or every two years for prevention of OP. Proper treatment with medications such as these can help people with OP live longer: In men younger than 60 and women younger than 75 who undergo treatment, life expectancy is increased by about 15 years compared to those who forgo treatment.[11]

Clinical scientists have revealed that suitable pharmaceutical education enhanced OP knowledge, personal satisfaction, and clinical fulfillment in post-menopausal osteoporotic women. A valid pharmaceutical-sponsored program incorporates a drug audit, training on OP, risk factors, and lifestyle adjustments, objectives of treatment, reactions, and the importance of medication adherence. Despite the effectiveness of medications in lowering the risk of bone fractures, poor adherence to treatment among patients is an issue in OP. Factors that impact well-being practices identified with OP include: (a) lack of information about OP, (b) lack of faith in the advantages of a particular treatment, (c) lack of motivation to overcome obstacles in OP treatment, (d) lack of social help, and (e) language barriers. Most effective mediations include more than one sort of intercession (e.g., instruction joined with self-administration) and utilization of techniques to impact patients' well-being convictions and frames of mind about OP and prescribed medications. Many analysts believe self-adequacy assumes a critical spot in sound practices for OP prevention as well as treatment adherence following diagnosis.[12]

Currently, the drugs that have been developed to treat or prevent OP may be used for:

- Those who have been diagnosed with OP
- Those who have low bone density (osteopenia)
- Those who are experiencing continued bone loss or fracture[13]

Medical practitioners have many options of drugs to choose from, depending on the condition of the individual patient:

- *Bisphosphonates.* These are the most commonly prescribed medications for OP. Bisphosphonates help to inhibit bone breakdown, preserve bone mass, and increase bone density in the hip and spine. These medications can be administered through pills or injection. In pill form, they may be taken either daily, weekly, or monthly, and by injection, they can be administered either once in a few months or once a year, depending on the composition of the drug. Bisphosphonates include:

- *Alendronate (Fosamax).* This is a class of bisphosphonate that acts as an inhibitor of osteoclast mediated bone resorption. It is a white, crystalline, nonhygroscopic powder that is soluble in water and slightly soluble in alcohol.

- *Risedronate (Actonel, Atelvia).* This is a bisphosphonate medication that helps in altering bone formation and breakdown, which slows down bone loss and prevents bone fractures. The drug is used to treat OP caused by menopause, steroid use, or gonadal failure.

- *Ibandronate (Boniva).* Like alendronate, ibandronate contains biosposphonates that inhibits osteoclast-mediated bone resorption. Boniva injection is delivered by intravenous administration only.

- *Zoledronic acid (Reclast, Zometa).* Just like other biosposphonate medicines, this helps in altering bone formation and breakdown and prevents bone fractures.

- *Teriparatide.* This is a drug that helps modify the body's parathyroid hormone, which plays a crucial role in bone remodeling and in maintaining the correct calcium balance in the bloodstream. It is the most recommended medicine for treating women and men with severe OP, including individuals who are at high risk of fracture and those who have not responded positively to other forms of medication. Teriparatide is taken through daily self-injection.

- *Denosumab.* This injectable medication falls within the class of medicines called RANKL inhibitors. It helps prevent bone loss by blocking receptors in the body to reduce bone breakdown. It is commonly used to treat OP in postmenopausal women as well as patients who do not respond well to other forms of medication. The drug is administered by injection every six months.

- *Raloxifene.* This drug belongs to a class of medicines known as SERMs. The drug functions just like the estrogen does on bone density in postmenopausal women. It helps slow down bone loss and also prevents spinal fracture.

- *Calcitonin.* This is a hormone produced in the thyroid gland. A synthetic form of this hormone, which helps in decelerating bone breakdown, is approved to treat postmenopausal OP, but not to prevent it. It is commonly administered as a nasal spray but can also be given as an injection.[14]

SURGICAL TREATMENT FOR OP

When other treatment methods such as exercise, medication, and diet fail, surgery may be the next option. Two minimally invasive surgical procedures are available to treat for osteoporotic fractures of the spine:

- *Kyphoplasty.* This surgery is designed to stop the pain caused by spinal fracture. It stabilizes bones and restores some or all of the lost vertebral body stature as a result of compression fracture.

- *Vertebroplasty.* This is a procedure whereby medical-grade cement is injected into the fractured vertebra to relieve back pain and restoring mobility. The surgery is mainly meant to stabilize vertebral compression fractures so as to stop their painful movement. This procedure is considered minimally invasive surgery because it is done through a small puncture in the skin instead of an open incision.[15]

STAYING ON COURSE WITH CONVENTIONAL OPTIONS

Taking OP treatment as prescribed can help prevent bone breaks and enables OP patients to remain mobile and independent. There are many successful treatment options available, but these can only work when taken as prescribed. Usually, patients with OP are open to taking medications, but many stop their treatment after just a year or so.

People with OP should consider medication routines (e.g., taking medicines each day before breakfast) that limit the effect on daily life. Patients can set reminders on a smartphone or other device to remind themselves to take their medicine or can post a note in a prominent place as a reminder. People with OP can also note important activities they have to remember to do in conjunction with receiving conventional treatment, including follow-up appointments. Organization can help patients plan for changes in life that will make it difficult for one to take medicine, for example, special events or gatherings.[16]

Patients can also ask family and friends to help them maintain their treatment plan. They can tell friends and family about their prescriptions and explain to them why it is vital to avoid breaking any bones. Osteoporosis patients can also talk about the challenges they are encountering with their doctor, who will be able to give advice on dealing with OP drugs and can present other treatment choices. It's important for individuals who have OP to contact local or online patient groups, where they can find emotional support and contact with others in similar circumstances.[17]

Another point to consider is that OP patients should not take any pain medications or supplements unless they are recommended by their doctor. These medications and supplements often have side effects such as dizziness, cough, and vomiting, which can cause fragility fractures. A surefire way of avoiding further fractures is to treat the cause of OP. The orthopedic surgeon can do a septoplasty to reduce the pain and aid mobility. It is important that OP patients take measures to maintain healthy bones, such as doing weight-bearing exercises and taking vitamin D and calcium supplements.[18]

ANALYSIS

Although OP cannot completely be reversed, the methods discussed here can greatly help in managing it. Unless advised otherwise by a medical practitioner, one should not solely rely on medication. The following practices should also be incorporated: exercise, healthy diet, smoking cessation, and limiting of alcohol intake.[19]

14

Lending a Helping Hand

THE USE OF SOCIAL MEDIA PLATFORMS FOR DIAGNOSIS AND MEDical advice is not recommended, but there is an advantage to sharing a personal experience. As the saying goes, "knowledge is power." Those who've suffered or are suffering from OP have a lot that they can share with their peers.[1]

HOW OP PATIENTS CAN HELP EACH OTHER

Patients can explain the initial stages of the disease and the symptoms that come along with the condition. This is usually firsthand information, from their own experience, which isn't normally available from medical practitioners. When patients engage their peers, they can tell whether they are in the initial or advanced mental stages of OP. They can explain how they manage the condition. This knowledge about how to handle a health condition is essential because the time a patient spends with the nurse or the doctor is minimal. Peers are very useful when it comes to guidance on how to manage a condition because one cannot constantly call doctors and nurses, day in and day out, for the smallest bits of advice.[2]

Peers are in a position to share the kinds of medication they have used or are using. They can also say (with disclaimers, of course) what has worked for them and what has not, noting any side effects of the medications they have used. Armed with this information, a patient can monitor their condition and can become very knowledgeable about treating and preventing OP. With every health condition there is a list of do's and don'ts, and that is also true in the case of OP. Peers can help in guiding patients about what to do, how to do it, and when to perform certain actions. They also guide patients on what to avoid, and when and why to avoid it. This knowledge can help patients have a much smoother healing journey.

Research has shown that patients in small communities of people with similar conditions usually find better health information, due to their exposure to different experiences, as compared to those patients going it alone. There is much more to the patient experience than a doctor or a nurse can convey because they haven't gone through the experience of suffering from OP. To many healthcare professionals, it is all just theories and studies (though credible) read in books. Information comes from fellow patients, it can help the newly diagnosed because they have already gone through it. This is information the doctor cannot provide. Peers can bring to light information that a doctor might not even be aware of.[3]

Peers can act as mentors in a patient's journey, as they are available to answer any direct questions regarding responses to medications. They walk with patients throughout the prescriptive period, from diagnosis to treatment to healing. They mentor patients on the do's and don'ts and can clarify information for newly diagnosed OP patients. Peer-provided information can guide new patients when preparing for their next appointment with the doctor since they, the peers, are already equipped with a lot of questions for the doctor.

When faced with a new health condition, it is not easy to synthesize all the information available online. The mountain of information out there might be intimidating, and at the same time, not everything posted online is correct. Therefore, information from an experienced community, explicitly passed from one individual to another, may be more reliable than information from websites with unknown sources.

Peers offer social and emotional support by encouraging each other. Observing other people's states of mind and body can be a wakeup call to living positively. Through peer interaction, new patients might find that they are better off than most, as their condition is not as severe as it is for their peers. Positive living is believed to have a significant contribution to the healing journey overall.[4]

Access to better healthcare is yet another advantage of peer-to-peer interaction. It is only through peers and medical professionals that one can get the best referrals to the medication, clinical care, and highly trained professionals. Engaging the right practitioners from the start makes the healing journey less bumpy and avoids constant referrals from one medical practitioner to the other. Hearing other people's stories and experiences can nudge patients into seeking expertise if similar experiences and symptoms make them suspect they may have the condition. Early diagnosis helps lessen the medical burden as the response to medication is usually faster than it would be when OP has reached an advanced stage. Another benefit of peer advice is that it comes at no cost. All that said, peer expertise should not be used in the absence of professional diagnosis and recommendation, because different people respond to treatment in different ways.[5]

Importance of Support Groups when Battling OP

People with OP do not have to enter the battle alone; they should look for connections and get help. How can they do this? Through support groups, of course. These groups bring together people who are going through or have already gone through similar experiences, giving patients and caregivers an opportunity to share personal experiences and firsthand information about OP, its treatment, coping strategies, and their feelings about it. There are a number of reasons why support groups in the struggle against OP are worth discussing, among them being the promotion of peer-based support. Support groups promote peer-based support by gathering people with OP together in a forum where they can interact with each other. Without support groups, it might be difficult to find people sharing the same experience. Support groups therefore play a pivotal role in bringing patients together to share their experiences and find companionship on their healing journey.[6]

Many people seek out support groups to help them gain more knowledge about their condition. They might want to know more about the symptoms, treatment, and management of OP. Many support groups offer newsletters that provide a deeper understanding of the condition explained in simple terms. There is usually a lot of information available online about various conditions, including OP, but patients should look for well-synthesized information. Support groups, both in-person and online, provide a source for reliable information and emotional assistance. When OP patients visit their doctor, often the only thing they get is clinical information and medication. Emotional support is not usually a part of that environment, but moral and emotional support are an integral part of the treatment.[7]

Studies have shown that individuals who receive moral and emotional support tend to heal faster than those who do not. Since this support is not always available in the hospitals, this is where the support groups come in. For people diagnosed with OP, or any chronic disease, managing the condition becomes a family concern. Through support networks, family members can be trained about the condition and how to manage it. Support groups also often offer newsletters and magazines to family members to help them understand the disease so they can better take care of their loved one.

Support groups also allow for practical treatment options. It is through support groups that patients can learn about the best options for treatment and the best local hospitals handling OP patients, as well as finding referrals to the best healthcare specialists. By sharing information, patients can find out which medications work best as well as which ones to avoid.

Support groups often offer seminars and training sessions for both OP patients and families. This gives the patients a deeper understanding of the disease. It can be a challenge to find professional training as an individual, but those services can be offered free of charge through support groups.

Support groups help patients gain a sense of empowerment and hope. As with many other chronic conditions, OP can impact mobility. In these cases, support groups are crucial, as they help empower people and give them hope for a brighter future. Through interaction with others, patients realize they are not going through this puzzling journey alone. There could be severe cases that persuade other OP sufferers to keep things going.[8]

Diagnosis with a chronic disease can cause a great deal of stress, anxiety, and depression, which can be exacerbated by loneliness and isolation. Support groups play a significant role in eliminating stress and depression by bringing patients together to share their experiences. It is on platforms such as these where the patients can drop all pretense about living with the condition and its pain and side effects. One goal of treatment is to stay motivated to manage OP and to stick to the medication plan. This can be tedious and difficult for some people. In some cases, patients do not show improvement despite prolonged medication, but support groups can help by encouraging them to stick to their treatment plan. Sharing progress with peers motivates patients to remain focused on their healing journey.[9]

For those who are immobile, online support groups provide emotional support and information about the symptoms, management, and treatment of OP. These groups often provide chat platforms where patients can directly connect with others. This gives them a sense of knowing they are not alone throughout the process. There's a certain level of satisfaction in being in a room—even a virtual one—with someone who understands you. Those suffering from any medical condition are better off in a place of empathy rather than pity, as compassion is a very powerful psychological device. Empathy empowers people to soldier on with practical experiences, while pity is just a transfer of guilt. Companions who have the same illness can offer specific motivation that no one else can provide.[10]

HOW CORPORATIONS CAN HELP IN THE BATTLE AGAINST OP

Osteoporosis is a disease that can affect anyone, anywhere, in both wealthy and developing nations. Once a person is affected, responsibility lands on the family, corporations, and the economy in general. Corporations are affected because some of their employees, or the family members of employees or executives, are OP patients. The impact of OP on the workforce, either directly or indirectly, in turn affects productivity, which has far-ranging effects on the economy. For this reason, corporations have roles in the fight against OP and other chronic diseases.

Research and development is one such role. It is the responsibility of pharmaceutical companies to manufacture medicine, so availability of medicines effective in preventing and treating OP depends on those companies. Their most significant role in the battle against OP and other chronic illnesses is to do research and develop drugs that can effectively cure these conditions. They should also ensure that there is sufficient supply of medicine, at a reasonable cost, so that it is available to those who need it.[11]

Strengthening the healthcare workforce is another role corporations play. Healthcare is the most sought-after service in every country in the world. Public hospitals are not in a position to handle the whole population, and this is where private corporations come in. Private-sector corporations help strengthen the clinical workforce by supporting the government and nongovernmental organizations (NGOs) through financing and strategic partnerships. In the fight against chronic diseases, these NGOs provide medical camps in the developing world where people go for free testing and treatment. They also contribute by opening hospitals, thus reducing the burden on the side of the government.[12]

At the operational level, corporations are responsible for providing insurance coverage to their employees. It is also their responsibility to ensure the health insurance they provide includes coverage for chronic disease prevention and management services. They should carry out health risk assessments on their employees to identify those who are affected by chronic medical conditions such as OP.[13]

Companies involved in manufacturing should ensure that the products they provide are healthy and, in the case of food products, safe for human consumption. This can be achieved by working in collaboration with the government, social meet-ups, and multilateral agencies. Studies have shown that most chronic diseases develop as a result of people's lifestyles, so it is the responsibility of corporations to produce healthy products that can improve quality of life. For instance, to counter the increase in cases of OP, food companies could produce products rich in calcium to promote bone health.[14]

Corporations have the ability to reach out to underserved populations on a massive scale. Marginalized communities are often disadvantaged when it comes to resource allocations pertaining to health and population demographics. In these cases, corporations can work to provide their products to the communities where they are needed most in a cost-effective, reliable, and timely manner.

To achieve this, companies can use the supply chain to reach out to underserved communities. In most cases, patients with chronic diseases in marginalized communities suffer silently, but corporate initiatives to reach out to them can help with prevention.

No single sector is solely responsible for health improvement, not even the government itself. Companies, however, can play a significant role in multisectoral partnerships. With valid partnerships, a greater population can be reached, significantly reducing the burden on the government. These partnerships also make it possible to offer critical health services at a considerably lower cost.[15]

A high level of corporate awareness is essential to success. Corporations should encourage health consciousness in their employees. Because of tight schedules at work, this can best be achieved through the creation of on-site wellness programs or by providing information through magazines or slide-show presentations. Employee training is essential as it is a way of reaching out to a larger population. Awareness of chronic diseases can play a great deal in prevention and regional disease control of OP. In terms of corporate social responsibility, corporations can go the extra mile to take care of vulnerable populations. Corporations can commit to supporting programs for caregivers of family members with OP and other chronic conditions as part of their corporate agenda. They can also sponsor free clinics for patients in marginalized areas.

Physical activity is essential for both physical and mental well-being. Corporations can promote physical activity by organizing or sponsoring marathons and other activities. These include communal events for both employees and the public. They can also start up gyms at the workplace for employees to use during their free time and encourage employees to walk or ride a bike to work instead of driving.

Corporations can do much more in the fight against chronic diseases and other ailments, but the most significant contribution remains in the research and development of medicine and technologies to diagnose, prevent, treat, and manage these conditions.[16]

HOW THE GOVERNMENT CAN HELP IN THE FIGHT AGAINST OP

Although no single sector is solely responsible for the healthcare status of a nation, the most significant burden rests with the government. It is the responsibility of government authorities in every country to provide affordable health services to its people. The role of the government in health involves prevention and control of epidemics. In the fight against OP, the top priority for the government is to carry out comprehensive clinical research to come up with the most efficient methods to eradicate the epidemic. The government can also support private sectors committed to research by financing or directly providing equipment required for research.[17]

Governments can establish an Osteoporosis Day in commemoration of the efforts put in place by governmental and nongovernmental institutions in the struggle against rising OP cases. This holiday would aim at initiating new strategies as well as implementing new programs. It would also be very helpful in raising awareness and spreading the message about OP. Government entities can partner with and lobby business owners to support OP programs, research, and education. Finances are usually the most significant problem for support groups. With financial support from the government, support groups can do great work in the fight against the epidemic. The government can also chip in by providing permits to hold meetings and gatherings aimed at bringing awareness to the public.[18]

Governments should equip hospitals with the proper equipment. When it comes to OP, DXA equipment is critical. These machines are costly, however, and without government intervention, many community and public hospitals may not have the resources to afford them. The government should also limit the exportation of used machines so they are available to purchase locally at a discounted rate. All of this supports the objective of providing affordable medical care.

It is the responsibility of the government of any region to provide affordable healthcare to its residents. This can be done by subsidizing the cost of medicine so that it is accessible to those with lower incomes. Since chronic diseases such as OP tend to be lifelong ailments, governments can provide universal medication coverage to reduce the financial burden on patients. Governments should also provide free vaccination to ensure that everyone is vaccinated against deadly viral epidemics. When it comes to viral diseases, which can worsen the already fragile health of people with OP and other chronic conditions, it is the role of federal and state governments to ensure that its citizens are well informed about any epidemic. Through its various agencies, the government can disseminate information about OP prevention and management. Government education sectors should also ensure that information about chronic diseases is integrated into the school curriculum in some way and should run awareness programs, rather than aimless criticism, on national media.[19]

Physical activities that have government backing help in promoting people's well-being. This is very important in fighting chronic diseases. Through its numerous departments, the government can develop and support programs to encourage and support healthy eating and regular physical activity. This can be done by ensuring healthy food is available in public vending machines and dining areas, and produced by food production plants. It is the responsibility of the government to work with stakeholders in food manufacturing and offer leadership in the prevention and control of OP and other chronic diseases. This can be achieved only through program and policy development, education, and development at both small and large scale.[20]

Governments can establish task forces or committees expected to meet regularly and design policies, which the government later reviews. They can observe progress on the implementation of wellness programs for those suffering from OP and other chronic conditions in order to appropriately identify problems and propose solutions. Task forces play a vital role in helping to propel government objectives forward. After programs related to chronic disease are integrated into the national development agenda, proper community-based planning will ensure there are enough resources allocated for large-scale programs, including those aimed at the marginalized communities discussed earlier. With adequate resources to fight the epidemic, it will be easier to address OP.[21]

ANALYSIS

In the final analysis, it is important to understand that most chronic diseases can be traced to lifestyle habits such as unhealthy dieting, tobacco use, physical inactivity, and the like. Government and corporations play a crucial role in reducing the risk of chronic diseases by implementing programs and policies make way for a healthy environment. Improved access to affordable OP-related healthcare is another topic that ought to be further explored in support groups.[22]

For Further Reading

Calton M, Calton J. *Rebuild Your Bones: The 12-Week Osteoporosis Protocol.* Rodale Books, 2019.

Daniels D. *Exercises for Osteoporosis, Third Edition: A Safe and Effective Way to Build Bone Density and Muscle Strength and Improve Posture and Flexibility.* Hatherleigh Press, 2008.

Gaby A. *Preventing and Reversing Osteoporosis: What You Can Do about Bone Loss—A Leading Expert's Natural Approach to Increasing Bone Mass.* Harmony, 1995.

Kearns A. *Mayo Clinic on Osteoporosis: Keep Your Bones Strong and Reduce Your Risk of Fractures.* Mayo Clinic Press, 2021.

Knopf K. *Beat Osteoporosis with Exercise: A Low-Impact Program for Building Strength, Increasing Bone Density and Improving Posture.* Ulysses Press, 2021.

Krusinski A, Astrom C, Sanford L, Brielyn J. *Gentle Yoga for Osteoporosis: A Safe and Easy Approach to Better Health and Well-Being through Yoga.* Hatherleigh Press, 2011.

McCormick RK. *The Whole-Body Approach to Osteoporosis: How to Improve Bone Strength & Reduce Your Fracture Risk.* New Harbinger Publications, 2009.

Nelson M, Wernick S. *Strong Women, Strong Bones: Everything You Need to Know to Prevent, Treat, and Beat Osteoporosis.* Tarcher Perigee, 2006.

Simpson L. *Dr. Lani's No-Nonsense Bone Health Guide. The Truth about Density Testing, Osteoporosis Drugs, and Building Bone Quality at Any Age.* Hunter House, 2014.

Wilen L, Wilen J. *Healing Remedies: More Than 1,000 Natural Ways to Relieve Common Ailments, from Arthritis and Allergies to Diabetes, Osteoporosis, and Many Others!* Ballantine Books, 2008.

Notes

Preface

1. Bonjour JP, Chevalley T, Ferrari S, Rizzoli R. The importance and relevance of peak bone mass in the prevalence of osteoporosis. *Salud Publica Mex.* 2009;51 Suppl 1:S5–17. Review.

2. Raisz LG. Pathogenesis of osteoporosis: concepts, conflicts, and prospects. *J Clin Invest.* 2005 Dec;115(12):3318–25.

3. Diab DL, Watts NB. Postmenopausal osteoporosis. *Curr Opin Endocrinol Diabetes Obes.* 2013 Dec;20(6):501–509; Goyal L, Goyal T, Gupta ND. Osteoporosis and periodontitis in postmenopausal women: a systematic review. *J Midlife Health.* 2017 Oct–Dec;8(4):151–58.

4. Jardí F, Laurent MR, Claessens F, Vanderschueren D. Estradiol and age-related bone loss in men. Physiol Rev. 2018 Jan 1; 98(1):1; Khosla S, Riggs BL. Pathophysiology of age-related bone loss and osteoporosis. *Endocrinol Metab Clin North Am.* 2005 Dec;34(4):1015–30, xi.

5. Kim CH, Chung CK, Kim MJ, Choi Y, Kim MJ, Hahn S, Shin S, Jung JM, Lee JH. Increased volume of lumbar surgeries for herniated intervertebral disc disease and cost-effectiveness analysis: a nationwide cohort study. *Spine (Phila Pa 1976).* 2017 Oct 31.

6. Dhaliwal R, Mikhail M, Usera G, Stolberg A, Islam S, Ragolia L, Aloia JF. The relationship of physical performance and osteoporosis prevention with vitamin D in older African Americans (PODA). *Contemp Clin Trials.* 2017 Dec 6; 65:39–45; Goode SC, Beshears JL, Goode RD, Wright TF, King A, Crist BD. Putting the brakes on breaks: osteoporosis screening and fracture prevention. *Geriatr Orthop Surg Rehabil.* 2017 Dec;8(4):238–43; Lems WF, Raterman HG. Critical issues and current challenges in osteoporosis and fracture prevention: an overview of unmet needs. *Ther Adv Musculoskelet Dis.* 2017 Dec; 9(12):299–316.

7. Sayed SA, Khaliq A, Mahmood A. Evaluating the risk of osteoporosis through bone mass density. *J Ayub Med Coll Abbottabad.* 2016 Oct–Dec;28(4):730–33.

8. Minett MM, Weidauer L, Wey HE, Binkley TL, Beare TM, Specker BL. Sports participation in high school and college leads to high bone density and greater rates of bone loss in young men: results from a population-based study. *Calcif Tissue Int.* 2018 Jan 4.

9. Lorenc R, Głuszko P, Franek E, Jabłoński M, Jaworski M, Kalinka-Warzocha E, Karczmarewicz E, Kostka T, Księzopolska-Orłowska K, Marcinowska-Suchowierska E, et al. Guidelines for the diagnosis and management of osteoporosis in Poland: update 2017. *Endokrynol Pol.* 2017; 68(5):604–609.

10. Anar C, Yüksel Yavuz M, Güldaval F, Varol Y, Kalenci D. Assessment of osteoporosis using the FRAX method and the importance of vitamin D levels in COPD patients. *Multidiscip Respir Med.* 2018 Jan 6;13:1.

11. Franek E, Wichrowska H, Gozdowski D, Puzianowska-Kuźnicka M. WHO fracture risk calculator (FRAX) in the assessment of obese patients with osteoporosis. *Endokrynol Pol.* 2009 Mar–Apr; 60(2):82–87.

CHAPTER 1

1. Schiedel F, Rödl R. Lower limb lengthening in patients with disproportionate short stature with achondroplasia: a systematic review of the last 20 years. *Disabil Rehabil.* 2012;34(12):982–87; Superti-Furga A, Unger S. Genetic disorders of bone—an historical perspective. *Bone.* 2017 Sep;102:1–4.

2. Figueras-Aloy J, Álvarez-Domínguez E, Pérez-Fernández JM, Moretones-Suñol G, Vidal-Sicart S, Botet-Mussons F. Metabolic bone disease and bone mineral density in very preterm infants. *J Pediatr.* 2014 Mar;164(3):499–504; Schulzke SM, Kaempfen S, Trachsel D, Patole SK. Physical activity programs for promoting bone mineralization and growth in preterm infants. *Cochrane Database Syst Rev.* 2014 Apr 22;(4):CD005387.

3. Battistuzzi PG. Röntgen and his discovery of "X-rays." *Ned Tijdschr Tandheelkd.* 2012 Feb;119(2):63; Sullivan PJ. Seeing the bones of things: a scan of X-rays' early history. *Can Fam Physician.* 2011 Oct;57(10):1174–75.

4. Ito A, Yajima A. Is bone biopsy necessary for the diagnosis of metabolic bone diseases? Necessity of bone biopsy. *Clin Calcium.* 2011 Sep;21(9):1388–92.

5. Stride PJ, Patel N, Kingston D. The history of osteoporosis: why do Egyptian mummies have porotic bones? *J R Coll Physicians Edinb.* 2013;43(3):254–61.

6. Androutsos G, Vladimiros L, Diamantis A. John Hunter (1728–1793): founder of scientific surgery and precursor of oncology. *J BUON.* 2007 Jul–Sep;12(3):421–27; Christen P, Ito K, Ellouz R, Boutroy S, Sornay-Rendu E, Chapurlat RD, van Rietbergen B. Bone remodelling in humans is load-driven but not lazy. *Nat Commun.* 2014 Sep;11(5):4855.

7. Hutchison RL, Rayan GM. Astley Cooper: his life and surgical contributions. *J Med Biogr.* 2015 Nov;23(4):209–16.

8. Uebelhart B, Uebelhart D. Epidemiology and treatment of osteoporosis in men. *Ther Umsch.* 2012 Mar;69(3):192–96.
9. Reifenstein EC Jr, Albright F. The classic: the metabolic effects of steroid hormones in osteoporosis. 1946. *Clin Orthop Relat Res.* 2011 Aug;469(8):2096–127.
10. Arabi A, Salamoun M, Ballout H, Fuleihan Gel-H. Densitometer type and impact on risk assessment for osteoporosis. *J Clin Densitom.* 2005 Fall; 8(3):261–66.
11. Vicente Molinero A, Lou Arnal S, Medina Orgaz E, Muñoz Jacobo S, Antonio Ibáñez Estrella J. Osteoporosis treatment with biphosphonates: approaches to care reality. *Aten Primaria.* 2011 Feb; 43(2):95–99.
12. [No authors listed]. Update on current care guidelines: osteoporosis. *Duodecim.* 2014;130(14):1466–68.
13. Brand RA. 50 years ago in CORR: the appearance of osteoporosis in ambulatory institutionalized males. Paul J. Vincent MD and Marshall R. Urist MD CORR 1961;19:245–52. *Clin Orthop Relat Res.* 2011 Jul; 469(7):2076–77.
14. Reginster JY, Burlet N. Osteoporosis: a still increasing prevalence. *Bone.* 2006 Feb;38(2 Suppl 1):S4–9.

CHAPTER 2

1. Rossignol M, Moride Y, Perreault S, Boivin JF, Ste-Marie LG, Robitaille Y, Poulin de Courval L, Fautrel B. Recommendations for the prevention of osteoporosis and fragility fractures: international comparison and synthesis. *Int J Technol Assess Health Care.* 2002 Summer;18(3):597–610.
2. Looker AC. Dysmobility syndrome and mortality risk in US men and women age 50 years and older. *Osteoporos Int.* 2015 Jan;26(1):93–102; Looker AC, Melton LJ 3rd, Harris TB, Borrud LG, Shepherd JA. Prevalence and trends in low femur bone density among older US adults: NHANES 2005–2006 compared with NHANES III. *J Bone Miner Res.* 2010 Jan;25(1):64–71.
3. Imerci A, Canbek U, Haghari S, Sürer L, Kocak M. Idiopathic juvenile osteoporosis: a case report and review of the literature. *Int J Surg Case Rep.* 2015;9:127–29.
4. Cauley JA. Defining ethnic and racial differences in osteoporosis and fragility fractures. *Clin Orthop Relat Res.* 2011 Jul;469(7):1891–1899.
5. Nguyen DN, O'Connell MB. Asian and Asian-American college students' awareness of osteoporosis. *Pharmacotherapy.* 2002 Aug;22(8):1047–54.
6. Miller RG, Ashar BH, Cohen J, Camp M, Coombs C, Johnson E, Schneyer CR. Disparities in osteoporosis screening between at-risk African-American and white women. *J Gen Intern Med.* 2005 Sep;20(9):847–51.
7. Evans KD, Taylor CA. Understanding osteoporosis prevalence in Hispanic women. *Radiol Technol.* 2006 Jul-Aug; 77(6):451–59; Yarbrough MM, Williams DP, Allen MM. Risk factors associated with osteoporosis in Hispanic women. *J Women Aging.* 2004; 16(3–4):91–104.

8. Holland A, Moffat T. Comparing measured calcium and vitamin D intakes with perceptions of intake in Canadian young adults: insights for designing osteoporosis prevention education. *Public Health Nutr.* 2017 Jul; 20(10):1760–67.

9. Viktoria Stein K, Dorner T, Lawrence K, Kunze M, Rieder A. Economic concepts for measuring the costs of illness of osteoporosis: an international comparison. *Wien Med Wochenschr.* 2009 May;159(9–10):253–61.

10. Kanis JA, McCloskey E, Branco J, Brandi ML, Dennison E, Devogelaer JP, Ferrari S, Kaufman JM, Papapoulos S, Reginster JY, Rizzoli R. Goal-directed treatment of osteoporosis in Europe. *Osteoporos Int.* 2014 Nov;25(11):2533–43.

11. Hopkins RB, Burke N, Von Keyserlingk C, Leslie WD, Morin SN, Adachi JD, Papaioannou A, Bessette L, Brown JP, Pericleous L, Tarride J. The current economic burden of illness of osteoporosis in Canada. *Osteoporos Int.* 2016 Oct;27(10):3023–32.

12. Morales-Torres J, Gutiérrez-Ureña S; Osteoporosis Committee of Pan-American League of Associations for Rheumatology. The burden of osteoporosis in Latin America. *Osteoporos Int.* 2004 Aug;15(8):625–32; Riera-Espinoza G. Epidemiology of osteoporosis in Latin America 2008. *Salud Publica Mex.* 2009;51 Suppl 1:S52–5.

13. Abd-Al-Atty MF. Regional fat, weight and osteoporosis in elderly women in Egypt. *East Mediterr Health J.* 2011 Nov;17(11):850–54; Keshtkar A, Tabatabaie O2,3, Matin N, Mohammadi Z, Ebrahimi M, Khashayar P, Asadi M. Clinical performance of seven prescreening tools for osteoporosis in Iranian postmenopausal women. *Rheumatol Int.* 2015 Dec;35(12):1995–2004.

14. Jeon YJ, Kim JW, Park JS. Factors associated with the treatment of osteoporosis in Korean postmenopausal women. *Women Health.* 2014;54(1):48–60.

15. Lai MM, Ang WM, McGuiness M, Larke AB. Undertreatment of osteoporosis in regional Western Australia. *Australas J Ageing.* 2012 Jun;31(2):110–14.

16. Reginster JY, Burlet N. Osteoporosis: a still increasing prevalence. *Bone.* 2006 Feb;38(2 Suppl 1):S4–9.

CHAPTER 3

1. Zhdan VM, Kitura OIe, Kitura IeM, Babanina MIu, Tkachenko MV. Treatment of postmenopausal osteoporosis in the general medical practice (clinical case). *Lik Sprava.* 2013 Mar;(2):85–89.

2. Jones JJ, Henry K. Early identification and treatment of osteoporosis in a rural internal medicine clinic: a quasi-experimental approach to quality improvement. *Orthop Nurs.* 2017 Mar/Apr; 36(2):147–52.

3. Watts NB, Bilezikian JP, Camacho PM, Greenspan SL, Harris ST, Hodgson SF, Kleerekoper M, Luckey MM, McClung MR, Pollack RP, Petak SM; AACE Osteoporosis Task Force. American Association of Clinical Endocrinologists Medical Guidelines for Clinical Practice for the diagnosis and

treatment of postmenopausal osteoporosis. *Endocr Pract.* 2010 Nov–Dec;16 Suppl 3:1–37.

4. Soybilgic A, Tesher M, Wagner-Weiner L, Onel KB. A survey of steroid-related osteoporosis diagnosis, prevention and treatment practices of pediatric rheumatologists in North America. *Pediatr Rheumatol Online J.* 2014 Jul 9;12:24.

5. Link TM. Osteoporosis imaging: state of the art and advanced imaging. *Radiology.* 2012 Apr;263(1):3–17; Link TM. Radiology of osteoporosis. *Can Assoc Radiol J.* 2016 Feb;67(1):28–40.

6. Kayan K, Kanis J, McCloskey E. Osteoporosis management by geriatricians in the UK. *Age Ageing.* 2003 Sep;32(5):553.

7. Atik OŞ. Has the awareness of orthopedic surgeons on osteoporosis been increased in the past decade? *Eklem Hastalik Cerrahisi.* 2015;26(2):63; Szklanny K, Kawik Ł, Kotela I. Osteoporosis in orthopedics—disease of civilization. *Przegl Lek.* 2010; 67(5):419–23.

8. Kasturi GC, Cifu DX, Adler RA. A review of osteoporosis: Part I. Impact, pathophysiology, diagnosis and unique role of the physiatrist. *PM R.* 2009 Mar;1(3):254–60.

9. Hirota T, Hirota K. Bone and nutrition: nutritional management of osteoporosis. *Clin Calcium.* 2015 Jul;25(7):1049–55.

10. Slomian J, Appelboom G, Ethgen O, Reginster JY, Bruyère O. Can new information and communication technologies help in the management of osteoporosis? *Womens Health (Lond).* 2014 May;10(3):229–32; Zhang Y, Liu P, Li J, Li K, Teng Y, Wang X, Li X. Communication factors-promising targets in osteoporosis treatment. *Curr Drug Targets.* 2014 Feb;15(2):156–63.

11. Beckerleg W, Oommen RA. Osteoporosis management in residential care: how internal and family medicine resident physicians translate evidence into practice. *Can Fam Physician.* 2017 May;63(5):411–12.

12. Beckerleg W, Oommen RA. Osteoporosis management in residential care: how internal and family medicine resident physicians translate evidence into practice. *Can Fam Physician.* 2017 May;63(5):411–12.

13. Field MH. Fractures, osteoporosis, and the endocrinologist. *Arch Intern Med.* 2003 Dec 8–22; 163(22):2796; Author reply 2796–97; Kurra S, Fink DA, Siris ES. Osteoporosis-associated fracture and diabetes. *Endocrinol Metab Clin North Am.* 2014 Mar;43(1):233–43.

14. Bernad Pineda M, González Fernández CM, Fernández Prada M, Fernández Campillo J, Maeso Martín R, Garcés Puentes MV. Rheumatology and osteoporosis (RETOSS): a vision of postmenopausal osteoporosis in rheumatology departments throughout Spain. *Reumatol Clin.* 2011 Jan–Feb;7(1):13–19.

15. Bennett DL, Post RD. The role of the radiologist when encountering osteoporosis in women. *AJR Am J Roentgenol.* 2011 Feb;196(2):331–37.

16. Gregersen M, Jensen NC, Mørch MM, Damsgaard EM. The effect of geriatric intervention on rehabilitation of elderly patients with hip fracture. *Ugeskr Laeger.* 2009 Nov 9;171(46):3336–40; Gregersen M, Mørch MM, Hougaard K, Damsgaard EM. Geriatric intervention in elderly patients with hip fracture in an orthopedic ward. *J Inj Violence Res.* 2012 Jul;4(2):45–51.

17. Farmer RP, Herbert B, Cuellar DO, et al. Osteoporosis and the orthopaedic surgeon: basic concepts for successful co-management of patients' bone health. *Int Orthop.* 2014 Aug; 38(8): 1731–38.

18. Kasturi GC, Cifu DX, Adler RA. A review of osteoporosis: Part I. Impact, pathophysiology, diagnosis and unique role of the physiatrist. *PM R.* 2009 Mar;1(3):254–60.

19. Martín Jiménez JA, Consuegra Moya B, Martín Jiménez MT. Nutritional factors in preventing osteoporosis. *Nutr Hosp.* 2015 Jul 18;32 Suppl 1:49–55.

20. Vytrisalova M, Touskova T, Fuksa L, Karascak R, Palicka V, Byma S, Stepan J. How general practitioners and their patients adhere to osteoporosis management: a follow-up survey among Czech general practitioners. *Front Pharmacol.* 2017; 8:258.

21. Roberto KA. Women with osteoporosis: the role of the family and service community. *Gerontologist.* 1988 Apr; 28(2):224–28.

22. Browner WS, Pressman AR, Nevitt MC, Cummings SR. Mortality following fractures in older women. The study of osteoporotic fractures. *Arch Intern Med.* 1996 Jul 22;156(14):1521–25; Leibson CL, Tosteson AN, Gabriel SE, Ransom JE, Melton LJ. Mortality, disability, and nursing home use for persons with and without hip fracture: A population-based study. *J Am Geriatr Soc.* 2002 Oct;50(10):1644–50; Magaziner J, Hawkes W, Hebel JR, Zimmerman SI, Fox KM, Dolan M, Felsenthal G, Kenzora J. Recovery from hip fracture in eight areas of function. *J Gerontol A Biol Sci Med Sci.* 2000;55(9):M498–507.

23. Melton LJ 3rd. Adverse outcomes of osteoporotic fractures in the general population. *J Bone Miner Res.* 2003 Jun;18(6):1139–41.

24. Chrischilles E, Shireman T, Wallace R. Costs and health effects of osteoporotic fractures. *Bone.* 1994 Jul-Aug;15(4):377–86.

25. Ettinger B, Black DM, Nevitt MC, Rundle AC, Cauley JA, Cummings SR, Genant HK, Genant HK. Contribution of vertebral deformities to chronic back pain and disability. The Study of Osteoporotic Fractures Research Group. *J Bone Miner Res.* 1992 Apr;7(4):449–56; Nevitt MC, Ettinger B, Black DM, Stone K, Jamal SA, Ensrud K, Segal M, Genant HK, Cummings SR. The association of radiographically detected vertebral fractures with back pain and function: a prospective study. *Ann Intern Med.* 1998 May 15;128(10):793–800; Ross PD. Clinical consequences of vertebral fractures. *Am J Med.* 1997 Aug 18;103(2A):30S–42S; Discussion 42S–43S.

26. Roh YH, Lee BK, Noh JH, Oh JH, Gong HS, Baek GH. Effect of anxiety and catastrophic pain ideation on early recovery after surgery for distal radius fractures. *J Hand Surg Am.* 2014 Nov;39(11):2258–64.e2.

27. Besser SJ, Anderson JE, Weinman J. How do osteoporosis patients perceive their illness and treatment? Implications for clinical practice. *Arch Osteoporos.* 2012;7:115–24.

28. Brainsky A, Glick H, Lydick E, Epstein R, Fox KM, Hawkes W, Kashner TM, Zimmerman SI, Magaziner J. The economic cost of hip fractures in community-dwelling older adults: a prospective study. *J Am Geriatr Soc.* 1997 Mar;45(3):281–87; Hoerger TJ, Downs KE, Lakshmanan MC, Lindroth RC, Plouffe L Jr, Wendling B, West SL, Ohsfeldt RL. Healthcare use among U.S. women aged 45 and older: total costs and costs for selected postmenopausal health risks. *J Womens Health Gend Based Med.* 1999 Oct;8(8):1077–89.

29. Brainsky A, Glick H, Lydick E, Epstein R, Fox KM, Hawkes W, Kashner TM, Zimmerman SI, Magaziner J. The economic cost of hip fractures in community-dwelling older adults: A prospective study. *J Am Geriatr Soc.* 1997 Mar;45(3):281–87.

CHAPTER 4

1. Radominski SC, Bernardo W, Paula AP, Albergaria BH, Moreira C, Fernandes CE, Castro CHM, Zerbini CAF, Domiciano DS, Mendonça LMC, Pompei LM, Bezerra MC, Loures MAR, Wender MCO, Lazaretti-Castro M, Pereira RMR, Maeda SS, Szejnfeld VL, Borba VZC. Brazilian guidelines for the diagnosis and treatment of postmenopausal OP. *Rev Bras Reumatol Engl Ed.* 2017;57 Suppl 2:452–66.

2. Glaser DL, Kaplan FS. OP. Definition and clinical presentation. *Spine (Phila Pa 1976).* 1997 Dec 15;22(24 Suppl):12S–16S.

3. Gambacciani M, Levancini M. Management of postmenopausal OP and the prevention of fractures. *Panminerva Med.* 2014 Jun;56(2):115–31.

4. Ettinger B, Black DM, Mitlak BH, Knickerbocker RK, Nickelsen T, Genant HK, Christiansen C, Delmas PD, Zanchetta JR, Stakkestad J, Glüer CC, Krueger K, Cohen FJ, Eckert S, Ensrud KE, Avioli LV, Lips P, Cummings SR. Reduction of vertebral fracture risk in postmenopausal women with OP treated with raloxifene: results from a 3-year randomized clinical trial. Multiple Outcomes of Raloxifene Evaluation (MORE) Investigators. *JAMA.* 1999 Aug 18;282(7):637–45.

5. Christianson MS, Shen W. OP prevention and management: nonpharmacologic and lifestyle options. *Clin Obstet Gynecol.* 2013 Dec;56(4):703–10.

6. Kennedy CC, Ioannidis G, Giangregorio LM, Adachi JD, Thabane L, Morin SN, Crilly RG, Marr S, Josse RG, Lohfeld L, Pickard LE, King S, van der Horst ML, Campbell G, Stroud J, Dolovich L, Sawka AM, Jain R, Nash L, Papaioannou A. An interdisciplinary knowledge translation intervention in long-term care: study protocol for the vitamin D and OP study (ViDOS) pilot cluster randomized controlled trial. *Implement Sci.* 2012 May 24;7:48.

7. St John IJ, Englund HM. Improving patient discharge education through daily educational bursts: a pilot study. *J Nurses Prof Dev.* 2020 Sep/Oct;36(5):283–87.

8. St John IJ, Englund HM. Improving patient discharge education through daily educational bursts: a pilot study. *J Nurses Prof Dev.* 2020 Sep/Oct;36(5):283–87.

9. Garnero P. The utility of biomarkers in OP management. *Mol Diagn Ther.* 2017 Aug;21(4):401–18.

10. Weaver CM, Alexander DD, Boushey CJ, Dawson-Hughes B, Lappe JM, LeBoff MS, Liu S, Looker AC, Wallace TC, Wang DD. Calcium plus vitamin D supplementation and risk of fractures: an updated meta-analysis from the National OP Foundation. *Osteoporos Int.* 2016 Jan;27(1):367–76.

11. Masterson J, Woodall T, Wilson CG, Ray L, Scott MA. Interprofessional care for patients with OP in a continuing care retirement community. *J Am Pharm Assoc.* (2003). 2016 Mar–Apr;56(2):184–88.

12. Yaşar E, Adigüzel E, Arslan M, Matthews DJ. Basics of bone metabolism and OP in common pediatric neuromuscular disabilities. *Eur J Paediatr Neurol.* 2018 Jan;22(1):17–26.

13. Kenny AM, Smith J, Noteroglu E, Waynik IY, Ellis C, Kleppinger A, Annis K, Dauser D, Walsh S. OP risk in frail older adults in assisted living. *J Am Geriatr Soc.* 2009 Jan;57(1):76–81.

14. Jachna CM, Whittle J, Lukert B, Graves L, Bhargava T. Effect of hospitalist consultation on treatment of OP in hip fracture patients. *Osteoporos Int.* 2003 Aug;14(8):665–71.

15. Al Amri A, Sadat-Ali M. Cancer chemotherapy-induced OP: how common is it among Saudi Arabian cancer survivors. *Indian J Cancer.* 2009 Oct–Dec;46(4):331–34.

16. Moayyeri A. The association between physical activity and osteoporotic fractures: a review of the evidence and implications for future research. *Ann Epidemiol.* 2008 Nov;18(11):827–35.

17. Pearson DA. Bone health and OP: the role of vitamin K and potential antagonism by anticoagulants. *Nutr Clin Pract.* 2007 Oct;22(5):517–44.

18. Jo WS, Cho EH, Kang BJ, et al. The impact of educational interventions on osteoporosis knowledge among Korean osteoporosis patients. *J Bone Metab.* 2018;25(2):115–21.

19. Solomon DH, Avorn J, Katz JN, Finkelstein JS, Arnold M, Polinski JM, Brookhart MA. Compliance with OP medications. *Arch Intern Med.* 2005 Nov 14;165(20):2414–19.

20. Bonura F. Prevention, screening, and management of OP: an overview of the current strategies. *Postgrad Med.* 2009 Jul;121(4):5–17.

21. Weycker D, Li X, Barron R, Bornheimer R, Chandler D. Hospitalizations for OP-related fractures: economic costs and clinical outcomes. *Bone Rep.* 2016 Jul 30;5:186–91.

22. Kelly RR, McDonald LT, Jensen NR, Sidles SJ, LaRue AC. Impacts of psychological stress on OP: clinical implications and treatment interactions. *Front Psychiatry.* 2019;10:200.

23. Costa AL, da Silva MA, Brito LM, Nascimento AC, do Carmo Lacerda Barbosa M, Batista JE, de Barros Bezerra GF, De Castro Viana GM, Filho WE, Vidal FC, Nascimento Mdo D. OP in primary care: an opportunity to approach risk factors. Rev Bras Reumatol Engl Ed. 2016 Mar–Apr;56(2):111–16.

CHAPTER 5

1. Hyassat D, Alyan T, Jaddou H, Ajlouni KM. Prevalence and risk factors of osteoporosis among Jordanian postmenopausal women attending the National Center for Diabetes, Endocrinology and Genetics in Jordan. *Biores Open Access.* 2017;6(1):85–93.

2. Notelovitz M. Androgen effects on bone and muscle. *Fertil Steril.* 2002 Apr;77 Suppl 4:S34–41.

3. Ogita M, Rached MT, Dworakowski E, Bilezikian JP, Kousteni S. Differentiation and proliferation of periosteal osteoblast progenitors are differentially regulated by estrogens and intermittent parathyroid hormone administration. *Endocrinology.* 2008;149(11):5713–23.

4. Cawthon PM. Gender differences in osteoporosis and fractures. *Clin Orthop Relat Res.* 2011 Jul;469(7):1900–1905.

5. Raisz LG. Pathogenesis of osteoporosis: concepts, conflicts, and prospects. *J Clin Invest.* 2005;115(12):3318–25.

6. Siddiqui JA, Partridge NC. Physiological bone remodeling: systemic regulation and growth factor involvement. *Physiology (Bethesda).* 2016;31(3):233–45.

7. Vierucci F, Saggese G, Cimaz R. Osteoporosis in childhood. *Curr Opin Rheumatol.* 2017 Sep;29(5):535–46.

8. Holm K, Hedricks C. Immobility and bone loss in the aging adult. *Crit Care Nurs Q.* 1989 Jun;12(1):46–51.

9. Hunter DJ, Sambrook PN. Bone loss. Epidemiology of bone loss. *Arthritis Res.* 2000;2(6):441–45.

10. Avdic D, Kapetanovic A. The influence of physical activity on the prevention of OP: the second congress of physical medicine and rehabilitation decors from Bosnia and Herzegovina with international participation. *Fojnica.* November 22–25,2007:61.

11. Heshmati HM, Khosla S. Idiopathic osteoporosis: a heterogeneous entity. *Ann Med Interne (Paris).* 1998 Mar;149(2):77–81.

12. Kelly HW, Van Natta ML, Covar RA, et al. Effect of long-term corticosteroid use on bone mineral density in children: a prospective longitudinal assessment in the childhood Asthma Management Program (CAMP) study. *Pediatrics.* 2008;122(1):e53–e61.

13. Delany AM, Dong Y, Canalis E. Mechanisms of glucocorticoid action in bone cells. *J Cell Biochem*. 1994 Nov;56(3):295–302.

14. Lodder MC, de Jong Z, Kostense PJ, Molenaar ET, Staal K, Voskuyl AE, Hazes JM, Dijkmans BA, Lems WF. Bone mineral density in patients with rheumatoid arthritis: relation between disease severity and low bone mineral density. *Ann Rheum Dis*. 2004 Dec;63(12):1576–80.

15. Ali T, Lam D, Bronze MS, Humphrey MB. Osteoporosis in inflammatory bowel disease. *Am J Med*. 2009 Jul;122(7):599–604.

16. Kärnsund S, Lo B, Bendtsen F, Holm J, Burisch J. Systematic review of the prevalence and development of osteoporosis or low bone mineral density and its risk factors in patients with inflammatory bowel disease. *World J Gastroenterol*. 2020 Sep 21;26(35):5362–74.

17. Khan TS, Fraser LA. Type 1 diabetes and osteoporosis: from molecular pathways to bone phenotype. *J Osteoporos*. 2015;2015:174186.

18. Ishimi Y. Osteoporosis and lifestyle. *J Nutr Sci Vitaminol (Tokyo)*. 2015;61 Suppl:S139–41.

19. Lewin E, Nielsen PK, Olgaard K. The calcium/parathyroid hormone concept of the parathyroid glands. *Curr Opin Nephrol Hypertens*. 1995 Jul;4(4):324–33.

20. Kanis JA, Johansson H, Johnell O, Oden A, De Laet C, Eisman JA, Pols H, Tenenhouse A. Alcohol intake as a risk factor for fracture. *Osteoporos Int*. 2005 Jul;16(7):737–42.

21. Yoon V, Maalouf NM, Sakhaee K. The effects of smoking on bone metabolism. *Osteoporos Int*. 2012 Aug;23(8):2081–92.

22. Benedetti MG, Furlini G, Zati A, Letizia Mauro G. The effectiveness of physical exercise on bone density in osteoporotic patients. *Biomed Res Int*. 2018 Dec 23;2018:4840531.

23. Borer KT. Physical activity in the prevention and amelioration of osteoporosis in women: interaction of mechanical, hormonal and dietary factors. *Sports Med*. 2005;35(9):779–830.

24. Sheweita SA, Khoshhal KI. Calcium metabolism and oxidative stress in bone fractures: Role of antioxidants. *Curr Drug Metab*. 2007 Jun;8(5):519–25.

25. Robbins J, Hirsch C, Whitmer R, Cauley J, Harris T. The association of bone mineral density and depression in an older population. *J Am Geriatr Soc*. 2001 Jun;49(6):732–36.

26. Lo JC, Kim S, Chandra M, Ettinger B. Applying ethnic-specific bone mineral density T-scores to Chinese women in the USA. *Osteoporos Int*. 2016 Dec;27(12):3477–84.

27. Mikuls TR, Saag KG, Curtis J, Bridges SL Jr, Alarcon GS, Westfall AO, Lim SS, Smith EA, Jonas BL, Moreland LW; CLEAR Investigators. Prevalence of osteoporosis and osteopenia among African Americans with early rheumatoid arthritis: the impact of ethnic-specific normative data. *J Natl Med Assoc*. 2005 Aug;97(8):1155–60.

28. Cauley JA, Chalhoub D, Kassem AM, Fuleihan Gel-H. Geographic and ethnic disparities in osteoporotic fractures. *Nat Rev Endocrinol.* 2014 Jun;10(6):338–51.

29. Sterling RS. Gender and race/ethnicity differences in hip fracture incidence, morbidity, mortality, and function. *Clin Orthop Relat Res.* 2011;469(7):1913–18.

30. Pouresmaeili F, Kamalidehghan B, Kamarehei M, Goh YM. A comprehensive overview on osteoporosis and its risk factors. *Ther Clin Risk Manag.* 2018;14:2029–49.

CHAPTER 6

1. Föger-Samwald U, Dovjak P, Azizi-Semrad U, Kerschan-Schindl K, Pietschmann P. Osteoporosis: Pathophysiology and therapeutic options. *EXCLI J.* 2020;19:1017–37.

2. Raisz LG. Pathogenesis of osteoporosis: concepts, conflicts, and prospects. *J Clin Invest.* 2005;115(12):3318–25.

3. Akkawi I, Zmerly H. Osteoporosis: current concepts. *Joints.* 2018;6(2):122–27.

4. Munch S, Shapiro S. The silent thief: osteoporosis and women's health care across the life span. *Health Soc Work.* 2006 Feb;31(1):44–53.

5. Llorente I, García-Castañeda N, Valero C, González-Álvaro I, Castañeda S. Osteoporosis in rheumatoid arthritis: dangerous liaisons. *Front Med (Lausanne).* 2020 Nov 23;7:601–18.

6. Dabas A, Malhotra R, Kumar R, Khadgawat R. Idiopathic juvenile osteoporosis in a child: a four-year follow-up with review of literature. *J Pediatr Endocrinol Metab.* 2021 Jul 30;34(11):1487–90.

7. Glaser DL, Kaplan FS. Osteoporosis: definition and clinical presentation. *Spine (Phila Pa 1976).* 1997 Dec 15;22(24 Suppl):12S–16S.

8. Giangregorio L, Papaioannou A, Cranney A, Zytaruk N, Adachi JD. Fragility fractures and the osteoporosis care gap: an international phenomenon. *Semin Arthritis Rheum.* 2006 Apr;35(5):293–305.

9. Kutsal FY, Ergin Ergani GO. Vertebral compression fractures: still an unpredictable aspect of osteoporosis. *Turk J Med Sci.* 2021;51(2):393–99.

10. Zhuang C, Wang Z, Chen W, Tian B, Li J, Lin H. Osteoporosis and endplate damage correlation using a combined approach of Hounsfield unit values and total endplate scores: a retrospective cross-sectional study. *Clin Interv Aging.* 2021;16:1275–83.

11. Xu W, Perera S, Medich D, Fiorito G, Wagner J, Berger LK, Greenspan SL. Height loss, vertebral fractures, and the misclassification of osteoporosis. *Bone.* 2011 Feb;48(2):307–11.

12. Sadat-Ali M, Al Elq AH, Al-Turki HA, Al-Mulhim FA, Al-Ali AK. Influence of vitamin D levels on bone mineral density and osteoporosis. *Ann Saudi Med.* 2011 Nov–Dec;31(6):602–608.

13. Westhovens R, Dequeker J. Rheumatoid arthritis and osteoporosis. *Z Rheumatol.* 2000;59 Suppl 1:33–38.

14. Phetfong J, Sanvoranart T, Nartprayut K, Nimsanor N, Seenprachawong K, Prachayasittikul V, Supokawej A. Osteoporosis: the current status of mesenchymal stem cell-based therapy. *Cell Mol Biol Lett.* 2016 Aug 12;21:12.

15. Lawrenson R, Nicholls P, Rivers-Latham R, Brown T, Barnardo J, Gray R. PIXI bone density screening for osteoporosis in postmenopausal women. *Maturitas.* 2006 Feb 20;53(3):245–51.

16. Wactawski-Wende J. Periodontal diseases and osteoporosis: association and mechanisms. *Ann Periodontol.* 2001 Dec;6(1):197–208.

17. Pillay I, Lyons D, German MJ, Lawson NS, Pollock HM, Saunders J, Chowdhury S, Moran P, Towler MR. The use of fingernails as a means of assessing bone health: a pilot study. *J Womens Health (Larchmt).* 2005 May;14(4):339–44.

18. Pillay I, Lyons D, German MJ, Lawson NS, Pollock HM, Saunders J, Chowdhury S, Moran P, Towler MR. The use of fingernails as a means of assessing bone health: a pilot study. *J Womens Health (Larchmt).* 2005 May;14(4):339–44.

19. Taniguchi Y, Makizako H, Kiyama R, Tomioka K, Nakai Y, Kubozono T, Takenaka T, Ohishi M. The association between osteoporosis and grip strength and skeletal muscle mass in community-dwelling older women. Int J Environ Res Public Health. 2019 Apr 6;16(7):1228.

20. Paolucci T, Saraceni VM, Piccinni G. Management of chronic pain in osteoporosis: challenges and solutions. *J Pain Res.* 2016;9:177–86.

21. Sinaki M, Brey RH, Hughes CA, Larson DR, Kaufman KR. Balance disorder and increased risk of falls in osteoporosis and kyphosis: significance of kyphotic posture and muscle strength. *Osteoporos Int.* 2005 Aug;16(8):1004–10.

22. Föger-Samwald U, Dovjak P, Azizi-Semrad U, Kerschan-Schindl K, Pietschmann P. Osteoporosis: Pathophysiology and therapeutic options. *EXCLI J.* 2020 Jul 20;19:1017–37.

CHAPTER 7

1. McCarthy EF. Genetic diseases of bones and joints. *Semin Diagn Pathol.* 2011 Feb;28(1):26–36.

2. Gayon J. From Mendel to epigenetics: history of genetics. *C R Biol.* 2016 Jul–Aug;339(7–8):225–30.

3. Laland KN, Odling-Smee J, Myles S. How culture shaped the human genome: bringing genetics and the human sciences together. *Nat Rev Genet.* 2010 Feb;11(2):137–48.

4. Wordsworth P. The influence of genetics in musculoskeletal diseases: a personal review of progress over 40 years. *Int J Rheum Dis.* 2019 Oct;22(10):1797–1802.

5. Albagha OM, Ralston SH. Genetics and osteoporosis. *Rheum Dis Clin North Am.* 2006;32(4):659–80.

6. Gregory D, Kaplan P, Scriver CR. Genetic causes of chronic musculoskeletal disease in childhood are common. *Am J Med Genet.* 1984 Nov;19(3):533–38.

7. Quayle J, Barakat A, Klasan A, Mittal A, Chan G, Gibbs J, Edmondson M, Stott P. Management of peri-prosthetic joint infection and severe bone loss after total hip arthroplasty using a long-stemmed cemented custom-made articulating spacer (CUMARS). *BMC Musculoskelet Disord.* 2021 Apr 16;22(1):358.

8. Sun P, He L, Jia K, et al. Regulation of body length and bone mass by Gpr126/Adgrg6. *Sci Adv.* 2020;6(12):eaaz0368.

9. Trajanoska K, Rivadeneira F. The genetic architecture of osteoporosis and fracture risk. *Bone.* 2019 Sep;126:2–10.

10. Kanis JA, Harvey NC, Cooper C, Johansson H, Odén A, McCloskey EV; Advisory Board of the National Osteoporosis Guideline Group. A systematic review of intervention thresholds based on FRAX: a report prepared for the National Osteoporosis Guideline Group and the International Osteoporosis Foundation. *Arch Osteoporos.* 2016 Dec;11(1):25.

11. Hallmayer J, Cleveland S, Torres A, Phillips J, Cohen B, Torigoe T, Miller J, Fedele A, Collins J, Smith K, Lotspeich L, Croen LA, Ozonoff S, Lajonchere C, Grether JK, Risch N. Genetic heritability and shared environmental factors among twin pairs with autism. *Arch Gen Psychiatry.* 2011 Nov;68(11):1095–102.

12. Yang TL, Shen H, Liu A, Dong SS, Zhang L, Deng FY, Zhao Q, Deng HW. A road map for understanding molecular and genetic determinants of osteoporosis. *Nat Rev Endocrinol.* 2020 Feb;16(2):91–103.

13. Harsløf T, Husted LB, Nyegaard M, Carstens M, Stenkjær L, Brixen K, Eiken P, Jensen JE, Børglum AD, Mosekilde L, Rejnmark L, Langdahl BL. Polymorphisms in the ALOX12 gene and osteoporosis. *Osteoporos Int.* 2011 Aug;22(8):2249–59.

14. Farhat GN, Cauley JA. The link between osteoporosis and cardiovascular disease. *Clin Cases Miner Bone Metab.* 2008;5(1):19–34.

15. Vimalraj S, Arumugam B, Miranda PJ, Selvamurugan N. Runx2: Structure, function, and phosphorylation in osteoblast differentiation. *Int J Biol Macromol.* 2015;78:202–208.

16. Dinarello CA. Proinflammatory cytokines. *Chest.* 2000 Aug;118(2):503–508.

17. Urano T, Inoue S. Genetics of osteoporosis. *Biochem Biophys Res Commun.* 2014 Sep 19;452(2):287–93.

CHAPTER 8

1. Dimitriou R, Jones E, McGonagle D, Giannoudis PV. Bone regeneration: current concepts and future directions. *BMC Med.* 2011;9:66.

2. McClung MR. The relationship between bone mineral density and fracture risk. *Curr Osteoporos Rep.* 2005 Jun;3(2):57–63.

3. Levis B, Benedetti A, Thombs BD; DEPRESsion Screening Data (DEPRESSD) Collaboration. Accuracy of Patient Health Questionnaire-9 (PHQ-9) for screening to detect major depression: individual participant data meta-analysis. *BMJ.* 2019 Apr 12;365:l1781.

4. Ionescu DF, Rosenbaum JF, Alpert JE. Pharmacological approaches to the challenge of treatment-resistant depression. *Dialogues Clin Neurosci.* 2015;17(2):111–26.

5. Ionescu DF, Rosenbaum JF, Alpert JE. Pharmacological approaches to the challenge of treatment-resistant depression. *Dialogues Clin Neurosci.* 2015;17(2):111–26.

6. Schatzberg AF. Treatment of severe depression with the selective serotonin reuptake inhibitors. *Depress Anxiety.* 1996–1997;4(4):182–89.

7. Ng QX, Venkatanarayanan N, Ho CY. Clinical use of Hypericum perforatum (St John's wort) in depression: a meta-analysis. *J Affect Disord.* 2017 Mar 1;210:211–21.

8. Thase ME. The role of monoamine oxidase inhibitors in depression treatment guidelines. *J Clin Psychiatry.* 2012;73 Suppl 1:10–16.

9. Davis LL, Ota A, Perry P, Tsuneyoshi K, Weiller E, Baker RA. Adjunctive brexpiprazole in patients with major depressive disorder and anxiety symptoms: an exploratory study. *Brain Behav.* 2016 Jul 24;6(10):e00520.

10. Mezuk B. Affective disorders, bone metabolism, and OP. *Clin Rev Bone Miner Metab.* 2008;6(3–4):101–13.

11. Rauma PH, Pasco JA, Berk M, et al. The association between major depressive disorder, use of antidepressants and bone mineral density (BMD) in men. *J Musculoskelet Neuronal Interact.* 2015;15(2):177–85.

12. Rauma PH, Koivumaa-Honkanen H, Williams LJ, Tuppurainen MT, Kröger HP, Honkanen RJ. Life satisfaction and bone mineral density among postmenopausal women: cross-sectional and longitudinal associations. *Psychosom Med.* 2014 Nov–Dec;76(9):709–15.

13. Pasco JA, Nicholson GC, Kotowicz MA. Cohort profile: Geelong OP Study. *Int J Epidemiol.* 2012 Dec;41(6):1565–75.

14. Oh EG, Lee JE, Yoo JY. A systematic review of the effectiveness of lifestyle interventions for improving bone health in women at high risk of OP. *JBI Libr Syst Rev.* 2012;10(30):1738–84.

15. Altindag O, Altindag A, Asoglu M, Gunes M, Soran N, Deveci Z. Relation of cortisol levels and bone mineral density among premenopausal women with major depression. *Int J Clin Pract.* 2007 Mar;61(3):416–20.

16. ltindag O, Altindag A, Asoglu M, Gunes M, Soran N, Deveci Z. Relation of cortisol levels and bone mineral density among premenopausal women with major depression. *Int J Clin Pract.* 2007 Mar;61(3):416–20.

17. Aguilar N. Counseling the patient with chronic illness: strategies for the health care provider. *J Am Acad Nurse Pract.* 1997 Apr;9(4):171–75.

18. Motyl KJ, Beauchemin M, Barlow D, et al. A novel role for dopamine signaling in the pathogenesis of bone loss from the atypical antipsychotic drug risperidone in female mice. *Bone.* 2017;103:168–76.

19. Xu G, Xiao Q, Zhou J, Wang X, Zheng Q, Cheng Y, Sun M, Li J, Liang F. Acupuncture and moxibustion for primary osteoporosis: an overview of systematic review. *Medicine (Baltimore).* 2020 Feb;99(9):e19334.

20. Kim J, Park E, An M. The cognitive impact of chronic diseases on functional capacity in community-dwelling adults. *J Nurs Res.* 2019 Feb;27(1):1–8.

21. Howard JT, Walick KS, Rivera JC. Preliminary evidence of an association between ADHD medications and diminished bone health in children and adolescents. *J Pediatr Orthop.* 2017 Jul/Aug;37(5):348–54.

22. Wippert PM, Rector M, Kuhn G, Wuertz-Kozak K. Stress and alterations in bones: an interdisciplinary perspective. *Front Endocrinol (Lausanne).* 2017 May;8:96.

23. Akkawi I, Zmerly H. OP: Current concepts. *Joints.* 2018;6(2):122–27.

24. Kostev K, Hadji P, Jacob L. Impact of OP on the risk of dementia in almost 60,000 patients followed in general practices in Germany. *J Alzheimers Dis.* 2018;65(2):401–407.

25. Frame G, Bretland KA, Dengler-Crish CM. Mechanistic complexities of bone loss in Alzheimer's disease: a review. *Connect Tissue Res.* 2020 Jan;61(1):4–18.

26. Yaffe K, Krueger K, Cummings SR, Blackwell T, Henderson VW, Sarkar S, Ensrud K, Grady D. Effect of raloxifene on prevention of dementia and cognitive impairment in older women: the Multiple Outcomes of Raloxifene Evaluation (MORE) randomized trial. *Am J Psychiatry.* 2005 Apr;162(4):683–90.

27. Robinson DM, Keating GM. Memantine: a review of its use in Alzheimer's disease. *Drugs.* 2006;66(11):1515–34.

28. Poirier J. Evidence that the clinical effects of cholinesterase inhibitors are related to potency and targeting of action. *Int J Clin Pract Suppl.* 2002 Jun;(127):6–19.

29. Robbins J, Hirsch C, Whitmer R, Cauley J, Harris T. The association of bone mineral density and depression in an older population. *J Am Geriatr Soc.* 2001 Jun;49(6):732–36.

CHAPTER 9

1. Estryn-Behar M, Kaminski M, Peigne E, Maillard MF, Pelletier A, Berthier C, Delaporte MF, Paoli MC, Leroux JM. Strenuous working conditions and musculo-skeletal disorders among female hospital workers. *Int Arch Occup Environ Health.* 1990;62(1):47–57.

2. Cizza G, Primma S, Coyle M, Gourgiotis L, Csako G. Depression and osteoporosis: a research synthesis with meta-analysis. *Horm Metab Res.* 2010;42(7):467–82.

3. Cizza G, Primma S, Coyle M, Gourgiotis L, Csako G. Depression and osteoporosis: a research synthesis with meta-analysis. *Horm Metab Res.* 2010;42(7):467–82.

4. Darragh AR, Sommerich CM, Lavender SA, Tanner KJ, Vogel K, Campo M. Musculoskeletal discomfort, physical demand, and caregiving activities in informal caregivers. *J Appl Gerontol.* 2015 Sep;34(6):734–60.

5. Huffman FG, Vaccaro JA, Zarini GG, Vieira ER. Osteoporosis, activities of daily living skills, quality of life, and dietary adequacy of congregate meal participants. *Geriatrics (Basel).* 2018 May;3(2):24.

6. Huffman FG, Vaccaro JA, Zarini GG, Vieira ER. Osteoporosis, activities of daily living skills, quality of life, and dietary adequacy of congregate meal participants. *Geriatrics (Basel).* 2018 May;3(2):24.

7. Lips P, van Schoor NM. Quality of life in patients with osteoporosis. *Osteoporos Int.* 2005 May;16(5):447–55.

8. Lips P, van Schoor NM. Quality of life in patients with osteoporosis. *Osteoporos Int.* 2005 May;16(5):447–55.

9. Alghadir AH, Gabr SA, Al-Eisa E. Physical activity and lifestyle effects on bone mineral density among young adults: sociodemographic and biochemical analysis. *J Phys Ther Sci.* 2015;27(7):2261–70.

10. Alghadir AH, Gabr SA, Al-Eisa E. Physical activity and lifestyle effects on bone mineral density among young adults: sociodemographic and biochemical analysis. *J Phys Ther Sci.* 2015;27(7):2261–70.

11. Resnick B, Nahm ES, Zhu S, et al. The impact of osteoporosis, falls, fear of falling, and efficacy expectations on exercise among community-dwelling older adults. *Orthop Nurs.* 2014;33(5):277–88.

12. Resnick B, Nahm ES, Zhu S, et al. The impact of osteoporosis, falls, fear of falling, and efficacy expectations on exercise among community-dwelling older adults. *Orthop Nurs.* 2014;33(5):277–88.

13. Conforti A, Chiamulera C, Moretti U, Colcera S, Fumagalli G, Leone R. Musculoskeletal adverse drug reactions: a review of literature and data from ADR spontaneous reporting databases. *Curr Drug Saf.* 2007 Jan;2(1):47–63.

14. Cizza G, Primma S, Coyle M, Gourgiotis L, Csako G. Depression and osteoporosis: a research synthesis with meta-analysis. *Horm Metab Res.* 2010 Jun;42(7):467–82.

15. Oleson CV, Busconi BD, Baran DT. Bone density in competitive figure skaters. *Arch Phys Med Rehabil.* 2002 Jan;83(1):122–28.

16. Cizza G, Primma S, Coyle M, Gourgiotis L, Csako G. Depression and osteoporosis: a research synthesis with meta-analysis. *Horm Metab Res.* 2010 Jun;42(7):467–82.

17. Barker KL, Javaid MK, Newman M, Minns Lowe C, Stallard N, Campbell H, Gandhi V, Lamb S. Physiotherapy Rehabilitation for Osteoporotic Vertebral Fracture (PROVE): Study protocol for a randomised controlled trial. *Trials*. 2014 Jan 14;15:22.

18. Feng Z, Zhan J, Wang C, Ma C, Huang Z. The association between musculoskeletal disorders and driver behaviors among professional drivers in China. *Int J Occup Saf Ergon*. 2020 Sep;26(3):551–61.

19. Lin YC, Fok LA, Schache AG, Pandy MG. Muscle coordination of support, progression and balance during stair ambulation. *J Biomech*. 2015 Jan 21;48(2):340–47.

20. Daneshmandi H, Choobineh A, Ghaem H, Karimi M. Adverse effects of prolonged sitting behavior on the general health of office workers. *J Lifestyle Med*. 2017;7(2):69–75.

21. Sinaki M. Exercise for patients with osteoporosis: management of vertebral compression fractures and trunk strengthening for fall prevention. *PM R*. 2012 Nov;4(11):882–88.

22. Huffman FG, Vaccaro JA, Zarini GG, Vieira ER. Osteoporosis, activities of daily living skills, quality of life, and dietary adequacy of congregate meal participants. *Geriatrics (Basel)*. 2018 May;3(2):24.

CHAPTER 10

1. Keen R. Osteoporosis: Strategies for prevention and management. *Best Pract Res Clin Rheumatol*. 2007 Feb;21(1):109–22.

2. Bauer UE, Briss PA, Goodman RA, Bowman BA. Prevention of chronic disease in the 21st century: elimination of the leading preventable causes of premature death and disability in the USA. *Lancet*. 2014 Jul 5;384(9937):45–52.

3. Shu AD, Stedman MR, Polinski JM, et al. Adherence to osteoporosis medications after patient and physician brief education: post hoc analysis of a randomized controlled trial. *Am J Manag Care*. 2009;15(7):417–24.

4. Siris ES, Miller PD, Barrett-Connor E, Faulkner KG, Wehren LE, Abbott TA, Berger ML, Santora AC, Sherwood LM. Identification and fracture outcomes of undiagnosed low bone mineral density in postmenopausal women: Results from the National Osteoporosis Risk Assessment. *JAMA*. 2001 Dec 12;286(22):2815–22.

5. Lane JM. Osteoporosis: medical prevention and treatment. *Spine (Phila Pa 1976)*. 1997 Dec 15;22(24 Suppl):32S–37S.

6. Rodan GA. Good hope for making osteoporosis a disease of the past. *Osteoporos Int*. 1994;4 Suppl 1:5–6.

7. Soen S, Usuba K, Crawford B, Adachi K. Family caregiver burden of patients with osteoporotic fracture in Japan. *J Bone Miner Metab*. 2021 Jul;39(4):612–22.

8. Price CT, Langford JR, Liporace FA. Essential nutrients for bone health and a review of their availability in the average North American diet. *Open Orthop J.* 2012;6:143–49.

9. Davies NJ. Improving self-management for patients with long-term conditions. *Nurs Stand.* 2010 Feb 24–Mar 2;24(25):49–56; quiz 58, 60.

10. Davies NJ. Improving self-management for patients with long-term conditions. *Nurs Stand.* 2010 Feb 24–Mar 2;24(25):49–56; quiz 58, 60.

11. Fini M, Salamanna F, Veronesi F, Torricelli P, Nicolini A, Benedicenti S, Carpi A, Giavaresi G. Role of obesity, alcohol and smoking on bone health. *Front Biosci (Elite Ed).* 2012 Jun 1;4:2586–606.

12. Wen HJ, Huang TH, Li TL, Chong PN, Ang BS. Effects of short-term step aerobics exercise on bone metabolism and functional fitness in postmenopausal women with low bone mass. *Osteoporos Int.* 2017 Feb;28(2):539–47.

13. Kelly RR, McDonald LT, Jensen NR, Sidles SJ, LaRue AC. Impacts of psychological stress on osteoporosis: clinical implications and treatment interactions. *Front Psychiatry.* 2019;10:200.

14. Lin J, Chen L, Ni S, Ru Y, Ye S, Fu X, Gan D, Li J, Zhang L, Han S, Zhu S. Association between sleep quality and bone mineral density in Chinese women vary by age and menopausal status. *Sleep Med.* 2019 Jan;53:75–80.

15. Cerroni AM, Tomlinson GA, Turnquist JE, Grynpas MD. Bone mineral density, osteopenia, and osteoporosis in the rhesus macaques of Cayo Santiago. *Am J Phys Anthropol.* 2000 Nov;113(3):389–410.

16. Francis RM, Selby PL. Osteomalacia. *Baillieres Clin Endocrinol Metab.* 1997 Apr;11(1):145–63.

17. Tournis S, Dede AD. Osteogenesis imperfecta—a clinical update. *Metabolism.* 2018 Mar;80:27–37.

18. Siris ES. Paget's disease of bone. *J Bone Miner Res.* 1998 Jul;13(7):1061–65.

19. Pai MV. Osteoporosis Prevention and Management. *J Obstet Gynaecol India.* 2017 Aug;67(4):237–42.

CHAPTER 11

1. Hong AR, Kim SW. Effects of resistance exercise on bone health. *Endocrinol Metab (Seoul).* 2018;33(4):435–44.

2. Oliveira MC, Vullings J, van de Loo FAJ. OP and osteoarthritis are two sides of the same coin paid for obesity. *Nutrition.* 2020 Feb;70:110486.

3. Resnick B, Nahm ES, Zhu S, et al. The impact of OP, falls, fear of falling, and efficacy expectations on exercise among community-dwelling older adults. *Orthop Nurs.* 2014;33(5):277–88.

4. Fujimoto K, Inage K, Orita S, et al. The nature of osteoporotic low back pain without acute vertebral fracture: a prospective multicenter study on the analgesic effect of monthly minodronic acid hydrate. *J Orthop Sci.* 2017 Jul;22(4):613–17.

5. Lewis RD, Modlesky CM. Nutrition, physical activity, and bone health in women. *Int J Sport Nutr.* 1998 Sep;8(3):250–84.

6. Ishikawa S, Kim Y, Kang M, Morgan DW. Effects of weight-bearing exercise on bone health in girls: a meta-analysis. *Sports Med.* 2013 Sep;43(9):875–92.

7. Ireland A, J Rittweger J. Exercise for OP: how to navigate between overeagerness and defeatism. *J Musculoskelet Neuronal Interact.* 2017;17(3):155–61.

8. Shanb AA, Youssef EF. The impact of adding weight-bearing exercise versus nonweight bearing programs to the medical treatment of elderly patients with OP. *J Family Community Med.* 2014;21(3):176–81.

9. Tankó LB, Christiansen C, Cox DA, Geiger MJ, McNabb MA, Cummings SR. Relationship between OP and cardiovascular disease in postmenopausal women. *J Bone Miner Res.* 2005 Nov;20(11):1912–20.

10. Kistler-Fischbacher M, Weeks BK, Beck BR. The effect of exercise intensity on bone in postmenopausal women (part 1): a systematic review. *Bone.* 2021 Feb;143:115696.

11. Wen HJ, Huang TH, Li TL, Chong PN, Ang BS. Effects of short-term step aerobics exercise on bone metabolism and functional fitness in postmenopausal women with low bone mass. *Osteoporos Int.* 2017 Feb;28(2):539–47.

12. Bean J, Herman S, Kiely DK, Callahan D, Mizer K, Frontera WR, Fielding RA. Weighted stair climbing in mobility-limited older people: a pilot study. *J Am Geriatr Soc.* 2002 Apr;50(4):663–70.

13. Potera C. Stretching the time between bone density screenings. *Am J Nurs.* 2012 Apr;112(4):15.

14. Wayne PM, Kiel DP, Krebs DE, Davis RB, Savetsky-German J, Connelly M, Buring JE. The effects of tai chi on bone mineral density in postmenopausal women: a systematic review. *Arch Phys Med Rehabil.* 2007 May;88(5):673–80.

15. Angın E, Erden Z, Can F. The effects of clinical pilates exercises on bone mineral density, physical performance and quality of life of women with postmenopausal osteoporosis. *J Back Musculoskelet Rehabil.* 2015;28(4):849–58.

16. Young CM, Weeks BK, Beck BR. Simple, novel physical activity maintains proximal femur bone mineral density, and improves muscle strength and balance in sedentary, postmenopausal Caucasian women. *Osteoporos Int.* 2007 Oct;18(10):1379–87.

17. Shanb AA, Youssef EF. The impact of adding weight-bearing exercise versus nonweight bearing programs to the medical treatment of elderly patients with osteoporosis. *J Family Community Med.* 2014;21(3):176–81.

18. Han L, Li SG, Zhai HW, Guo PF, Chen W. Effects of weight training time on bone mineral density of patients with secondary osteoporosis after hemiplegia. *Exp Ther Med.* 2017 Mar;13(3):961–65.

19. Harding AT, Beck BR. Exercise, osteoporosis, and bone geometry. *Sports (Basel).* 2017;5(2):29.

20. Mishra N, Mishra VN, Devanshi. Exercise beyond menopause: dos and don'ts. *J Midlife Health*. 2011;2(2):51–56.

21. Elliott TLP, Marshall KS, Lake DA, Wofford NH, Davies GJ. The effect of sitting on stability balls on nonspecific lower back pain, disability, and core endurance: a randomized controlled crossover study. *Spine (Phila Pa 1976)*. 2016 Sep 15;41(18):E1074–E1080.

22. Benedetti MG, Furlini G, Zati A, Letizia Mauro G. The effectiveness of physical exercise on bone density in osteoporotic patients. *Biomed Res Int*. 2018;2018:4840531.

23. Mosti MP, Kaehler N, Stunes AK, Hoff J, Syversen U. Maximal strength training in postmenopausal women with osteoporosis or osteopenia. *J Strength Cond Res*. 2013 Oct;27(10):2879–86.

24. Liang MT, Quezada L, Lau WJ, Sokmen B, Spalding TW. Effect of short-term upper-body resistance training on muscular strength, bone metabolic markers, and BMD in premenopausal women. *Open Access J Sports Med*. 2012;3:201–208.

25. Jang JH, Jee YS, Oh HW. Frequency-effect of playing screen golf on body composition and golf performance in middle-aged men. *J Exerc Rehabil*. 2014;10(5):271–78.

26. Kunutsor SK, Leyland S, Skelton DA, et al. Adverse events and safety issues associated with physical activity and exercise for adults with osteoporosis and osteopenia: a systematic review of observational studies and an updated review of interventional studies. *J Frailty Sarcopenia Falls*. 2018;3(4):155–78.

27. Kunutsor SK, Leyland S, Skelton DA, et al. Adverse events and safety issues associated with physical activity and exercise for adults with osteoporosis and osteopenia: a systematic review of observational studies and an updated review of interventional studies. *J Frailty Sarcopenia Falls*. 2018;3(4):155–78.

28. Iwamoto J, Takeda T, Sato Y, Uzawa M. Effect of whole-body vibration exercise on lumbar bone mineral density, bone turnover, and chronic back pain in post-menopausal osteoporotic women treated with alendronate. *Aging Clin Exp Res*. 2005 Apr;17(2):157–63.

29. Vlachopoulos D, Barker AR, Ubago-Guisado E, Williams CA, Gracia-Marco L. The effect of a high-impact jumping intervention on bone mass, bone stiffness and fitness parameters in adolescent athletes. *Arch Osteoporos*. 2018;13(1):128.

30. Pettersson U, Alfredson H, Nordström P, Henriksson-Larsén K, Lorentzon R. Bone mass in female cross-country skiers: relationship between muscle strength and different BMD sites. *Calcif Tissue Int*. 2000 Sep;67(3):199–206.

31. Todd JA, Robinson RJ. Osteoporosis and exercise. *Postgrad Med J*. 2003;79(932):320–23.

CHAPTER 12

1. Muñoz-Garach A, García-Fontana B, Muñoz-Torres M. Nutrients and dietary patterns related to osteoporosis. *Nutrients.* 2020;12(7):1986.

2. Locke A, Schneiderhan J, Zick SM. Diets for health: goals and guidelines. *Am Fam Physician.* 2018 Jun 1;97(11):721–28.

3. Zuckerman-Levin N, Hochberg Z, Latzer Y. Bone health in eating disorders. *Obes Rev.* 2014 Mar;15(3):215–23.

4. Zuckerman-Levin N, Hochberg Z, Latzer Y. Bone health in eating disorders. *Obes Rev.* 2014 Mar;15(3):215–23.

5. Saeg F, Orazi R, Bowers GM, Janis JE. Evidence-based nutritional interventions in wound care. *Plast Reconstr Surg.* 2021 Jul 1;148(1):226–38.

6. Ahmadieh H, Arabi A. Vitamins and bone health: beyond calcium and vitamin D. *Nutr Rev.* 2011 Oct;69(10):584–98.

7. Nair R, Maseeh A. Vitamin D: The "sunshine" vitamin. *J Pharmacol Pharmacother.* 2012;3(2):118–26.

8. Brondani JE, Comim FV, Flores LM, Martini LA, Premaor MO. Fruit and vegetable intake and bones: a systematic review and meta-analysis. *PLoS One.* 2019 May 31;14(5):e0217223.

9. Laird E, Molloy AM, McNulty H, Ward M, McCarroll K, Hoey L, Hughes CF, Cunningham C, Strain JJ, Casey MC. Greater yogurt consumption is associated with increased bone mineral density and physical function in older adults. *Osteoporos Int.* 2017 Aug;28(8):2409–19.

10. Bonjour JP, Schürch MA, Rizzoli R. Proteins and bone health. *Pathol Biol (Paris).* 1997 Jan;45(1):57–59.

11. Nirmala FS, Lee H, Kim JS, Jung CH, Ha TY, Jang YJ, Ahn J. Fermentation improves the preventive effect of soybean against bone loss in senescence-accelerated mouse prone 6. *J Food Sci.* 2019 Feb;84(2):349–57.

12. Riva A, Togni S, Giacomelli L, Franceschi F, Eggenhoffner R, Feragalli B, Belcaro G, Cacchio M, Shu H, Dugall M. Effects of a curcumin-based supplementation in asymptomatic subjects with low bone density: a preliminary 24-week supplement study. *Eur Rev Med Pharmacol Sci.* 2017 Apr;21(7):1684–89.

13. Shen CL, Yeh JK, Cao JJ, Wang JS. Green tea and bone metabolism. *Nutr Res.* 2009 Jul;29(7):437–56. Erratum in: *Nutr Res.* 2009 Sep;29(9):684.

14. Prentice A. Diet, nutrition and the prevention of osteoporosis. *Public Health Nutr.* 2004 Feb;7(1A):227–43.

15. Ogur R, Uysal B, Ogur T, Yaman H, Oztas E, Ozdemir A, Hasde M. Evaluation of the effect of cola drinks on bone mineral density and associated factors. *Basic Clin Pharmacol Toxicol.* 2007 May;100(5):334–38.

16. Promislow JH, Goodman-Gruen D, Slymen DJ, Barrett-Connor E. Retinol intake and bone mineral density in the elderly: the Rancho Bernardo Study. *J Bone Miner Res.* 2002 Aug;17(8):1349–58.

17. Galland L. Diet and inflammation. *Nutr Clin Pract.* 2010 Dec;25(6):634–40.

18. Carbone L, Johnson KC, Huang Y, et al. Sodium intake and osteoporosis. findings from the Women's Health Initiative. *J Clin Endocrinol Metab.* 2016;101(4):1414–21.

19. Maurel DB, Boisseau N, Benhamou CL, Jaffre C. Alcohol and bone: review of dose effects and mechanisms. *Osteoporos Int.* 2012 Jan;23(1):1–16.

20. Zhou J, Ma YH, Zhou Z, Chen Y, Wang Y, Gao X. Intestinal absorption and metabolism of epimedium flavonoids in osteoporosis rats. *Drug Metab Dispos.* 2015 Oct;43(10):1590–600.

21. Tian L, Yu X. Fat, sugar, and bone health: a complex relationship. *Nutrients.* 2017 May 17;9(5):506.

22. Nakayama K, Katayama S. Osteoporosis and intake of carbohydrates. *Clin Calcium.* 2005 Apr;15(4):680–83.

23. Nakayama K, Katayama S. Osteoporosis and intake of carbohydrates. *Clin Calcium.* 2005 Apr;15(4):680–83.

24. Wachman A, Bernstein DS. Diet and osteoporosis. *Lancet.* 1968 May 4;1(7549):958–59.

CHAPTER 13

1. Wang T, Liu Q, Tjhioe W, Zhao J, Lu A, Zhang G, Tan RX, Zhou M, Xu J, Feng HT. Therapeutic potential and outlook of alternative medicine for osteoporosis. *Curr Drug Targets.* 2017;18(9):1051–68.

2. Banu J, Varela E, Fernandes G. Alternative therapies for the prevention and treatment of osteoporosis. *Nutr Rev.* 2012 Jan;70(1):22–40.

3. Leung PC, Siu WS. Herbal treatment for osteoporosis: a current review. *J Tradit Complement Med.* 2013 Apr;3(2):82–87.

4. Pan H, Jin R, Li M, Liu Z, Xie Q, Wang P. The effectiveness of acupuncture for osteoporosis: a systematic review and meta-analysis. *Am J Chin Med.* 2018;46(3):489–513.

5. Saetung S, Chailurkit LO, Ongphiphadhanakul B. Thai traditional massage increases biochemical markers of bone formation in postmenopausal women: a randomized crossover trial. *BMC Complement Altern Med.* 2013;13:69.

6. Bervoets DC, Luijsterburg PA, Alessie JJ, Buijs MJ, Verhagen AP. Massage therapy has short-term benefits for people with common musculoskeletal disorders compared to no treatment: a systematic review. *J Physiother.* 2015 Jul;61(3):106–16.

7. Kennedy AB, Cambron JA, Sharpe PA, Travillian RS, Saunders RP. Process for massage therapy practice and essential assessment. *J Bodyw Mov Ther.* 2016 Jul;20(3):484–96.

8. Iolascon G, Moretti A, Toro G, Gimigliano F, Liguori S, Paoletta M. Pharmacological therapy of osteoporosis: what's new? *Clin Interv Aging.* 2020 Mar 26;15:485–91.

9. Skjødt MK, Frost M, Abrahamsen B. Side effects of drugs for osteoporosis and metastatic bone disease. *Br J Clin Pharmacol.* 2019 Jun;85(6):1063–71.

10. Abrahamsen B. Adverse effects of bisphosphonates. *Calcif Tissue Int.* 2010 Jun;86(6):421–35.

11. Watts NB. Bisphosphonate treatment of osteoporosis. *Clin Geriatr Med.* 2003 May;19(2):395–414.

12. Vidal M, Thibodaux RJ, Neira LFV, Messina OD. Osteoporosis: a clinical and pharmacological update. *Clin Rheumatol.* 2019 Feb;38(2):385–95

13. Vidal M, Thibodaux RJ, Neira LFV, Messina OD. Osteoporosis: a clinical and pharmacological update. *Clin Rheumatol.* 2019 Feb;38(2):385–95.

14. Tu KN, Lie JD, Wan CKV, et al. Osteoporosis: a review of treatment options. *P T.* 2018;43(2):92–104.

15. Chandra RV, Maingard J, Asadi H, Slater LA, Mazwi TL, Marcia S, Barr J, Hirsch JA. Vertebroplasty and kyphoplasty for osteoporotic vertebral fractures: what are the latest data? *AJNR Am J Neuroradiol.* 2018 May;39(5):798–806.

16. Sözen T, Özışık L, Başaran NÇ. An overview and management of osteoporosis. *Eur J Rheumatol.* 2017;4(1):46–56.

17. Gold DT. The nonskeletal consequences of osteoporotic fractures: psychologic and social outcomes. *Rheum Dis Clin North Am.* 2001 Feb;27(1):255–62.

18. Catalano A, Martino G, Morabito N, Scarcella C, Gaudio A, Basile G, Lasco A. Pain in osteoporosis: from pathophysiology to therapeutic approach. *Drugs Aging.* 2017 Oct;34(10):755–65.

19. Wang T, Liu Q, Tjhioe W, Zhao J, Lu A, Zhang G, Tan RX, Zhou M, Xu J, Feng HT. Therapeutic potential and outlook of alternative medicine for osteoporosis. *Curr Drug Targets.* 2017;18(9):1051–68.

CHAPTER 14

1. Kloseck M, Fitzsimmons DA, Speechley M, Savundranayagam MY, Crilly RG. Improving the diagnosis and treatment of osteoporosis using a senior-friendly peer-led community education and mentoring model: a randomized controlled trial. *Clin Interv Aging.* 2017;12:823–33.

2. Kloseck M, Fitzsimmons DA, Speechley M, Savundranayagam MY, Crilly RG. Improving the diagnosis and treatment of osteoporosis using a senior-friendly peer-led community education and mentoring model: a randomized controlled trial. *Clin Interv Aging.* 2017;12:823–33.

3. Nahm ES, Resnick B, Brown C, et al. The effects of an online theory-based bone health program for older adults. *J Appl Gerontol.* 2017;36(9):1117–44.

4. Doull M, O'Connor AM, Welch V, Tugwell P, Wells GA. Peer support strategies for improving the health and well-being of individuals with chronic diseases. *Cochrane Database Syst Rev.* 2017;2017(6):CD005352.

5. Doull M, O'Connor AM, Welch V, Tugwell P, Wells GA. Peer support strategies for improving the health and well-being of individuals with chronic diseases. *Cochrane Database Syst Rev.* 2017;2017(6):CD005352.

6. Davison KP, Pennebaker JW, Dickerson SS. Who talks? The social psychology of illness support groups. *Am Psychol*. 2000 Feb;55(2):205–17.

7. Turner J, Kelly B. Emotional dimensions of chronic disease. *West J Med*. 2000;172(2):124–28.

8. Doull M, O'Connor AM, Welch V, Tugwell P, Wells GA. Peer support strategies for improving the health and well-being of individuals with chronic diseases. *Cochrane Database Syst Rev*. 2017;2017(6):CD005352.

9. Kumano H. Osteoporosis and stress. *Clin Calcium*. 2005 Sep;15(9):1544–47.

10. Cohen M, Quintner J, Buchanan D, Nielsen M, Guy L. Stigmatization of patients with chronic pain: the extinction of empathy. *Pain Med*. 2011 Nov;12(11):1637–43.

11. Nickel S, von dem Knesebeck O. Effectiveness of community-based health promotion interventions in urban areas: A systematic review. *J Community Health*. 2020 Apr;45(2):419–34.

12. Gellert GA. Non-governmental organizations in international health: past successes, future challenges. *Int J Health Plann Manage*. 1996 Jan–Mar;11(1):19–31.

13. Song Z, Baicker K. Effect of a workplace wellness program on employee health and economic outcomes: a randomized clinical trial. *JAMA*. 2019 Apr 16;321(15):1491–501.

14. Goodridge D, Bandara T, Marciniuk D, et al. Promoting chronic disease management in persons with complex social needs: a qualitative descriptive study. *Chron Respir Dis*. 2019;16:1479973119832025.

15. Goodridge D, Bandara T, Marciniuk D, et al. Promoting chronic disease management in persons with complex social needs: a qualitative descriptive study. *Chron Respir Dis*. 2019;16:1479973119832025.

16. Molnár E, Mahmood A, Ahmad N, Ikram A, Murtaza SA. The interplay between corporate social responsibility at employee level, ethical leadership, quality of work life and employee pro-environmental behavior: the case of healthcare organizations. *Int J Environ Res Public Health*. 2021 Apr 24;18(9):4521.

17. Raphael D, Brown I, Bryant T, Wheeler J, Herman R, Houston J, Hussain M, Lanphier C, Lightfoot B, McClelland B, McIntosh B, Stevens I, Weisbeck F. How government policy decisions affect seniors' quality of life: findings from a participatory policy study carried out in Toronto, Canada. *Can J Public Health*. 2001 May–Jun;92(3):190–95.

18. Tang N, Eisenberg JM, Meyer GS. The roles of government in improving health care quality and safety. *Jt Comm J Qual Saf*. 2004 Jan;30(1):47–55.

19. Tang N, Eisenberg JM, Meyer GS. The roles of government in improving health care quality and safety. *Jt Comm J Qual Saf*. 2004 Jan;30(1):47–55.

20. Gelius P, Messing S, Goodwin L, Schow D, Abu-Omar K. What are effective policies for promoting physical activity? A systematic review of reviews. *Prev Med Rep*. 2020;18:101095.

21. Gjerris A. Sharing the responsibilities: the roles of the government. *Int Clin Psychopharmacol.* 1999 Jun;14 Suppl 3:S7–S9.

22. Hiswåls AS, Hamrin CW, Vidman Å, Macassa G. Corporate social responsibility and external stakeholders' health and wellbeing: s viewpoint. *J Public Health Res.* 2020;9(1):1742.

Index

About the Author

NAHEED ALI, MD, PHD, IS A PHYSICIAN BY EDUCATION AND A professional writer by choice since 2005. He brings more than 15 years of experience working in a remote environment. Now a digital nomad, he currently freelances as a health and wellness writer by way of HealthcarePropulsion.com.